Atlas of OCULOFACIAL RECONSTRUCTION

Principles and Techniques for the Repair of Periocular Defects

Atlas of
OCULOFACIAL
RECONSTRUCTION

Principles and Techniques for the Repair of Periocular Defects

GERALD J. HARRIS, MD, FACS

Professor of Ophthalmology
Chief, Orbital and Oculoplastic Surgery
Medical College of Wisconsin

EDITOR-IN-CHIEF:
Ophthalmic Plastic and Reconstructive Surgery

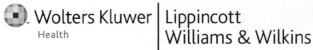

Wolters Kluwer Health | Lippincott Williams & Wilkins

Senior Executive Editor: Jonathan W. Pine, Jr.
Managing Editor: Molly M. Ward
Marketing Manager: Lisa Parry
Production Editor: Beth Martz
Design Coordinator: Stephen Druding
Compositor: Cadmus Communications, a Cenveo company

351 West Camden Street   530 Walnut Street
Baltimore, MD 21201   Philadelphia, PA 19106

Printed in China

9 8 7 6 5 4 3 2 1

Library of Congress Cataloging-in-Publication Data

Harris, Gerald J.
  Atlas of oculofacial reconstruction : principles and techniques for the repair of periocular defects / Gerald J. Harris.
    p. ; cm.
  Includes bibliographical references and index.
  ISBN-13: 978-0-7817-9651-4
  ISBN-10: 0-7817-9651-2
  1. Eye-sockets—Surgery—Atlases. 2. Ophthalmic plastic surgery—Atlases. I. Title.
  [DNLM: 1. Ophthalmologic Surgical Procedures—methods—Atlases. 2. Face—surgery—Atlases. 3. Reconstructive Surgical Procedures—methods—Atlases. WW 17 H314a 2009]
  RD527.E94H37 2009
  617.7′80592—dc22   2008050206

DISCLAIMER

Care has been taken to confirm the accuracy of the information present and to describe generally accepted practices. However, the authors, editors, and publisher are not responsible for errors or omissions or for any consequences from application of the information in this book and make no warranty, expressed or implied, with respect to the currency, completeness, or accuracy of the contents of the publication. Application of this information in a particular situation remains the professional responsibility of the practitioner; the clinical treatments described and recommended may not be considered absolute and universal recommendations.

The authors, editors, and publisher have exerted every effort to ensure that drug selection and dosage set forth in this text are in accordance with the current recommendations and practice at the time of publication. However, in view of ongoing research, changes in government regulations, and the constant flow of information relating to drug therapy and drug reactions, the reader is urged to check the package insert for each drug for any change in indications and dosage, and for added warnings and precautions. This is particularly important when the recommended agent is a new or infrequently employed drug.

Some drugs and medical devices presented in this publication have Food and Drug Administration (FDA) clearance for limited use in restricted research settings. It is the responsibility of the health care provider to ascertain the FDA status of each drug or device planned for use in their clinical practice.

To purchase additional copies of this book, call our customer service department at **(800) 638-3030** or fax orders to **(301) 223-2320**. International customers should call **(301) 223-2300**.

Visit Lippincott Williams & Wilkins on the Internet: http://www.lww.com. Lippincott Williams & Wilkins customer service representatives are available from 8:30 am to 6:00 pm, EST.

Dedication

To my wife, Susan, and my sons, Michael and David

Preface

Youthful perspectives drive innovation in all areas of medicine. There is also something to be said for a seasoned viewpoint, particularly when one surgeon presumes to advise others in matters of technique. In a 30-year career, technical details are conceived or adopted, modified, refined, and sometimes discarded. Adjustments are continually made in response to outcomes in thousands of cases that vary in subtle ways. Reporting a single-surgeon experience may have its limitations, but it also "controls" for the operator variable in that technical evolution.

This atlas addresses the reconstruction of eyelid and oculofacial defects after tissue removal or loss. Despite the specific focus, the wide variety of defects and their functional and aesthetic implications require a full volume to discuss management in necessary detail. Somewhat more than a hundred case studies are included, and I have tried to faithfully reproduce flap design and transposition by superimposing graphics on operative photographs, rather than relying on artists' interpretations. The atlas is divided into chapters according to *oculofacial sector,* and the anatomic concerns specific to each sector are addressed with tailored surgical procedures. A final section deals with issues common to all areas.

The text is intended to improve aesthetic and functional outcomes in these challenging cases. I hope that it will find a home on the reader's desktop (real or virtual), and will repeatedly serve as a resource when patients present with defects of unanticipated size or complexity.

Gerald J. Harris, MD, FACS

Acknowledgments

I thank Deb Wahlers, desktop publishing specialist and computer guru, for her help converting 500-odd figure parts into print-worthy TIFF files. Others who contributed through the years to the surgery represented herein include all of my esteemed fellows, as well as my operating room technicians—particularly, Mary Beier, Unis Matthews, and Jeanne Powers. The experience reported would not have been possible without the 18-year collaboration of Marcelle Neuburg, MD, Chief of Dermatologic Surgery at the Medical College of Wisconsin.

The time devoted to this project had to be stolen from somewhere, and for that I thank Vikki Jimenez, my secretary; Hollis Brunner, Managing Editor, *Ophthalmic Plastic and Reconstructive Surgery*; and Susan Harris, my understanding and supportive wife.

Last, I thank Jonathan Pine, Senior Executive Editor, Lippincott Williams & Wilkins, for shepherding the text through the publication process.

Contents

Oculofacial Reconstruction: Current Challenges

*T*he reconstruction of periocular defects following definitive tumor excision or tissue-loss trauma can have significant visual and aesthetic consequences. Surgical outcomes for these defects—both within and beyond the orbital perimeter—can affect the unique anatomy and dynamic action of the eyelids and eyebrows. In recent years, a rising incidence of facial skin cancer and the increasing impact of Mohs micrographic surgery have influenced periocular reconstruction in both number and kind, creating new challenges for oculoplastic and other facial reconstructive surgeons. This growing experience affords the opportunity to develop a systematic approach to oculofacial reconstruction.

More than one million new cases of nonmelanoma skin cancer, mainly basal cell carcinoma, are diagnosed and treated annually in the United States.[1] One in six individuals will be affected at some point, and the incidence is increasing. More than 80% of lesions involve the head and neck. Historically, many methods have been used to treat nonmelanomatous skin cancer, but Mohs micrographic surgery is increasingly perceived as yielding the highest cure rates while maximally conserving normal tissue. The American College of Mohs Surgery reports 5-year cure rates of 99% for previously untreated tumors and 95% for recurrences.[2]

The Mohs procedure, generally performed by fellowship-trained dermatologic surgeons, should be differentiated from standard resection with frozen-section control. Although both methods rely on frozen-section monitoring, the Mohs technique is distinguished by beveled excision and flattening of the specimen, which allow the entire periphery and base to be examined simultaneously.[3] More than 60 fellowship programs (most are 1 year in duration) are recognized by the Mohs society.[2] Training includes micrographic excision, dermatopathology, and reconstructive techniques. Depending on defect size and location, however, Mohs surgeons frequently enlist other specialists for repairs. In addition to increasing efficiency for all physicians involved, the division of labor encourages complete tumor excision that is not inhibited by reconstructive concerns.

Patients introduced to this surgical collaboration after first presenting to their ophthalmologists are likely to have eyelid margin lesions and corresponding full-thickness defects (Fig. 1.1). Patients who first present to dermatologists generally have more peripheral, nonmarginal lesions and skin/muscle defects (Figs. 1.2 and 1.3). In these cases, the eyelid margins are not involved by tumor, but reconstructive outcomes can affect them, and appreciation of periocular anatomy and dynamics is critical in surgical repair.

Mohs surgery patients may have failed prior standard surgery or radiation, may have had multiple primary facial cancers through the years, and may have severely sun-damaged skin—all of which can limit skin elasticity and reconstructive options. Defects after Mohs excision vary widely in size, shape, and depth, and repair choices range from simple grafts to a variety of

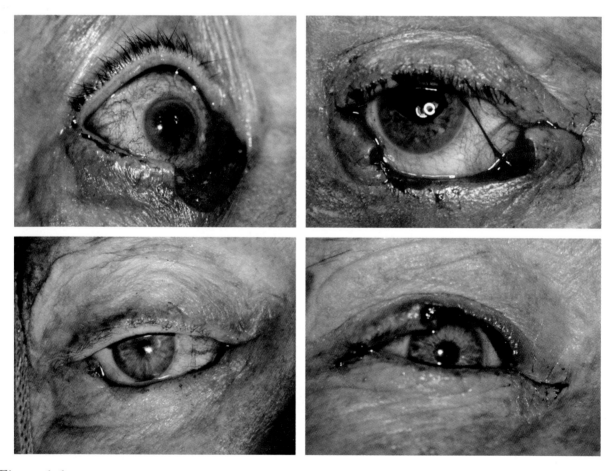

Figure 1.1

Full-thickness eyelid margin defects after Mohs resection of basal cell carcinomas.

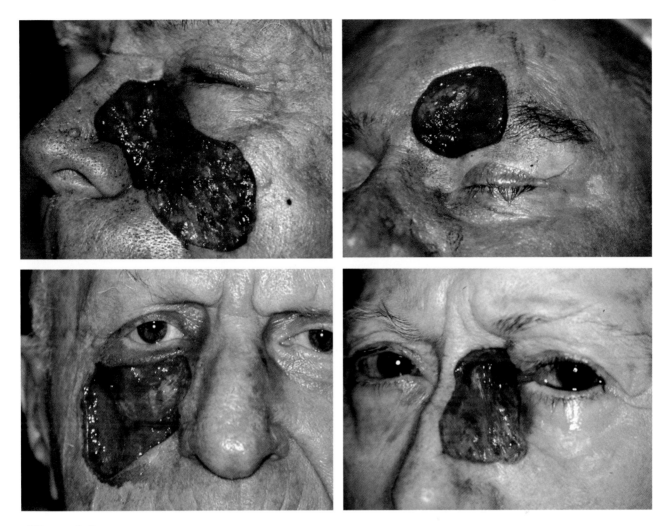

Figure 1.2

Nonmarginal oculofacial defects after Mohs surgery. (Modified and reproduced with permission from Lippincott Williams & Wilkins. Sources: Harris GJ, Perez N. Anchored flaps in post-Mohs reconstruction of the lower eyelid, cheek, and lateral canthus: avoiding eyelid distortion. Ophthal Plast Reconstr Surg 2003;19:5–13. Harris GJ, Logani SC. Multiple aesthetic unit flaps for medial canthal reconstruction. Ophthal Plast Reconstr Surg 1998;14:352–359. Harris GJ, Garcia GH. Advancement flaps for large defects of the eyebrow, glabella, forehead and temple. Ophthal Plast Reconstr Surg 2002;18:138–145.)

flaps. There are "many ways to skin a cat," and each surgeon finds what works best for him or her. This atlas respectfully offers personal lessons learned in more than 30 years of periocular reconstruction.

Some recurrent themes underlie the procedures described: The eyelids, canthal angles, and eyebrows are mobile and therefore vulnerable to the non-directed pull of wound bed contraction. Facial skin is a passive envelope, subject to deep attachments and traction vectors. Anchoring of oculofacial

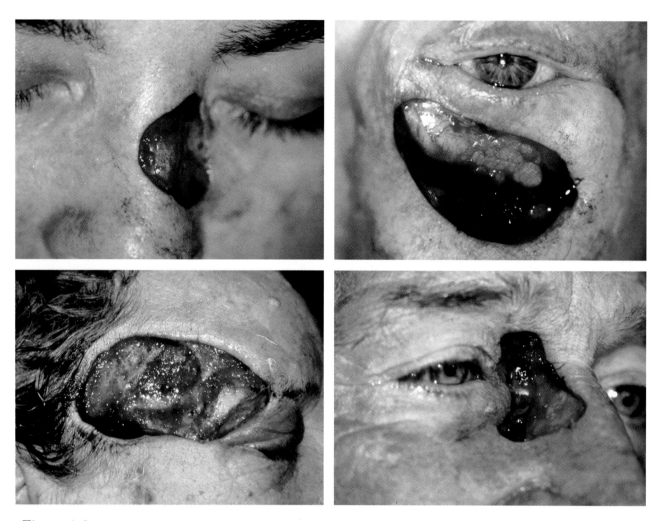

Figure 1.3

Nonmarginal oculofacial defects after Mohs surgery. (Modified and reproduced with permission from Lippincott Williams & Wilkins. Sources: Harris GJ, Logani, SC. Multiple aesthetic unit flaps for medial canthal reconstruction. Ophthal Plast Reconstr Surg 1998;14:352–359. Harris GJ, Garcia GH. Advancement flaps for large defects of the eyebrow, glabella, forehead and temple. Ophthal Plast Reconstr Surg 2002;18:138–145.)

flaps to underlying, fixed tissue can stretch the skin to our advantage, while limiting distortion of the periocular tissues.

In oculofacial reconstruction, defect size matters, but location may be more important. Therefore, the surgical principles in each region apply to defects of varied magnitude. Marginal, full-thickness defects require restoration of the bilamellar eyelid architecture. More peripheral, nonmarginal defects throughout the upper two thirds of the face potentially affect eyelid or eyebrow position, and we can divide this oculocentric area into a few broad sectors, each with distinct anatomic concerns (Fig. 1.4).

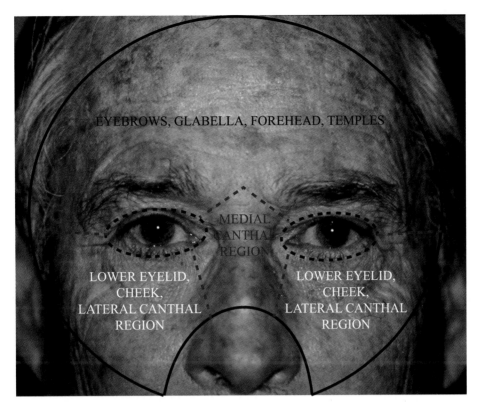

EYEBROWS, GLABELLA, FOREHEAD, TEMPLES

MEDIAL CANTHAL REGION

LOWER EYELID, CHEEK, LATERAL CANTHAL REGION

LOWER EYELID, CHEEK, LATERAL CANTHAL REGION

Figure 1.4

Sectorial approach to the repair of nonmarginal oculofacial defects. Specific anatomic concerns in each area inform reconstructive decisions.

Using this regional approach, I primarily address reconstruction after tumor resection. Because the final tumor-free defect is often not predictable from a lesion's clinical appearance, the reconstructive challenge may be unknown until the patient presents for the actual repair. The surgeon must therefore have a broad range of options readily at hand, and it is hoped that this atlas will repeatedly serve as a practical guide at those times. With minor modifications, the principles and techniques can be applied to posttraumatic reconstruction as well. The bulk of the text is devoted to surgical details that differ among the oculofacial sectors. The final chapter addresses issues of preoperative counseling, operative instrumentation, and postoperative management common to all areas. I presuppose that readers of this book have a basic knowledge of eyelid anatomy, but key relationships are emphasized when pertinent. Cadaver-based anatomic depictions and detailed to-scale diagrams can be found in several excellent manuals of orbital anatomy and oculoplastic surgery-texts of broader focus.[4–7]

References

1. American Cancer Society. What are the key statistics about squamous and basal cell skin cancer? Available at: www.cancer.org/docroot/CRI/content/CRI_2_4_1X_What_are_the_key_statistics_for_skin_cancer_51.asp?rnav=cri. Accessed July 30, 2007.
2. Mohs College. About Mohs micrographic surgery. Available at: www.mohscollege.org/AboutMMS.html. Accessed July 30, 2007.
3. Bowen GM, White GL, Gerwels JW. Mohs micrographic surgery. Am Fam Physician 2005;72:845–848.
4. Zide BM, Jelks GW. Surgical Anatomy of the Orbit. New York: Raven Press, 1985.
5. Zide BM. Surgical Anatomy around the Orbit: The System of Zones. Philadelphia: Lippincott Williams & Wilkins, 2006.
6. Dutton JJ, Waldrop TG. Atlas of Clinical and Surgical Orbital Anatomy. Philadelphia: WB Saunders, 1994.
7. Wobig JL, Dailey RA. Oculofacial Plastic Surgery. New York: Thieme, 2004.

Marginal Eyelid Defects

*F*or maintenance of normal vision, full-thickness marginal defects require the restoration of normal eyelid architecture and function. The eyelids affect vision through their resting levels, range of movement, apposition to the globe, and specialized anatomic features.

Complete opening maximizes the field of vision; complete closure protects the globe from injury and desiccation (Fig. 2.1). Dynamic excursion between those extremes—blinking—distributes the tear film across the cornea and propels tears into the lacrimal drainage apparatus. Proper function requires eyelid-to-globe apposition, which depends on adequate horizontal tension and balanced vertical forces on internal and external surfaces (Fig. 2.2).

Conjunctival elements that interface with the cornea include a nonkeratinizing epithelium, mucin-secreting goblet cells, and aqueous fluid-producing accessory lacrimal glands. Oil-secreting Meibomian glands within the densely fibrous tarsal plates discharge at the eyelid margins, completing the trilaminar (mucin–water–oil) tear film (Figs. 2.3 and 2.4). Eyelash continuity protects the eyes from particulate debris, and normal eyelash direction prevents corneal irritation. The multiple, histologically distinct layers of the eyelid are each thin and tightly adherent at the eyelid margin. For practical purposes, the marginal eyelids can be considered bilamellar: tarsoconjunctiva, posteriorly; skin–muscle (with negligible intervening substantia propria), anteriorly.

Considering the unique features and functions of the eyelids, the preferred techniques of reconstruction involve maximal use of residual eyelid tissue before resorting to other sources. If a defect is too large for approximation of the remaining full-thickness marginal tissue, bilamellar reconstruction requires transfer of tarsoconjunctiva (from the same eyelid, the ipsilateral opposing eyelid, or a contralateral eyelid) and surfacing with thin skin (as a flap or graft). Other mucosally surfaced tissue (e.g., hard palate mucosa) should replace the posterior lamella only if sufficient tarsoconjunctiva is unavailable. Transposed or grafted tissues must be positioned within the defect with appropriate regard to horizontal tension and vertical forces.

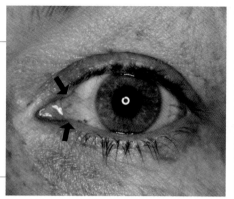
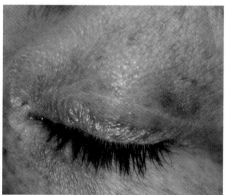

Figure 2.1

Normal eyelid position and excursion afford unimpeded vision, globe protection, and tear distribution across the palpebral fissure and toward the lacrimal puncta (arrows).

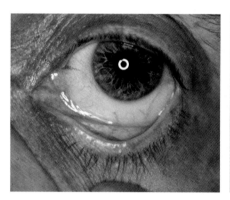
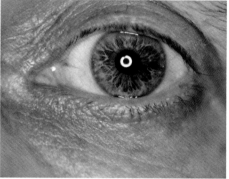

Figure 2.2

Elasticity of the tarsal plates and their fibrous attachments allows the eyelids to move over and conform to the convex surface of the eye. Release of manual distraction should be followed by rapid reapposition, which depends on adequate horizontal tension in the tarsoligamentous sling and orbicularis muscle, as well as balanced vertical forces on anterior and posterior layers.

Although there are many surgeon-specific modifications and preferences, the reconstruction of full-thickness marginal defects generally involves established techniques applied in a size-related progression. However, the assignment of techniques based on specific millimeter measurements or percentage widths cannot be rigid, because the distensibility of residual tissues varies in individual cases. In addition, that distensibility can be increased by relaxing canthal attachments through a broad range. A "laddered" approach considers defect size relative to tissue elasticity, and is built on the conversion of an irregular marginal defect to a pentagon, which is directly approximated. Adjunctive relaxing procedures, dictated by tissue tension, may include lateral cantholysis, cantholysis + titrated orbital septum release, and cantholysis + orbital septum release + semicircular rotation flap. Marginal defects beyond the limits of the foregoing are converted to rectangles and are repaired with a

Figure 2.3

A smooth, moist conjunctival surface depends on a nonkeratinized epithelial layer containing goblet cells, a normally functioning main lacrimal gland, accessory lacrimal glands in the conjunctival fornices, and Meibomian glands (whitish vertical stripes) within the fibrous tarsal plates.

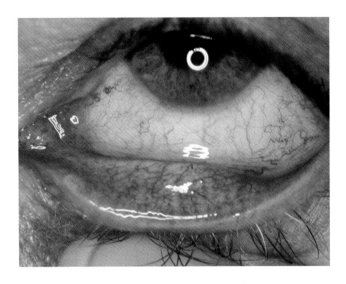

Figure 2.4

The Meibomian glands open on the conjunctival aspect of the eyelid margin, appearing as white dots (white arrow). The "gray line" (black arrow) marks the mucocutaneous junction. The eyelashes emanate from the cutaneous aspect (yellow arrow) and are directed away from the globe.

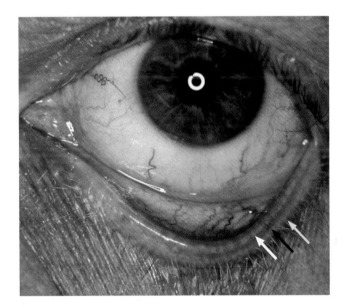

tarsoconjunctival flap + a skin flap or graft, or with a free tarsal graft + a skin or myocutaneous flap.

Technique selection and surgical details are best described with representative cases. Procedures applicable to the lower eyelid are depicted in Figures 2.5 to 2.49.

Figure 2.5

A. Mohs defects of the eyelid margin begin as saucer-shaped excisions of anterior lamellar tumors. As such, they are not uniform with respect to anatomic planes. Histographically directed deeper level excisions are more focal, adding to defect irregularity.
B. Direct repair requires conversion to a pentagonal defect, and begins with parallel vertical incisions and amputation of any residual tarsus (white lines). **C.** Because of differences in their elasticity, the more inferior tissues are excised as triangles of slightly decreasing size from superficial to deep layers: skin (yellow-black lines), orbicularis muscle (orange-black lines), and septum/retractors/conjunctiva (green-black lines). For simplicity, full-thickness pentagonal resections are designated with single yellow or yellow-black lines in the figure drawings that follow.

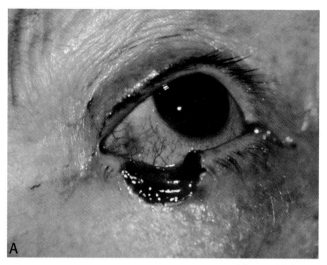

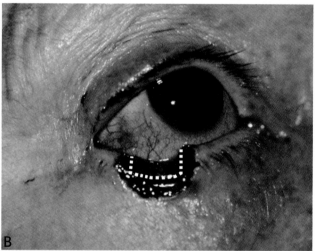

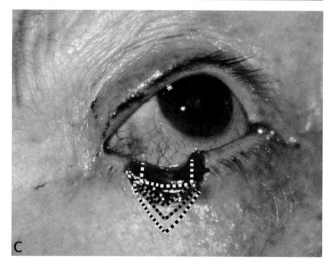

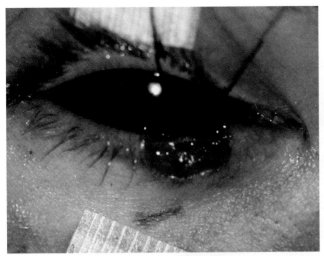
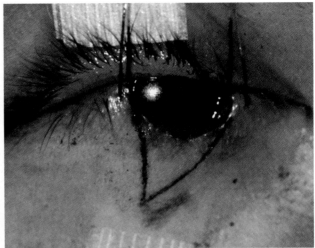
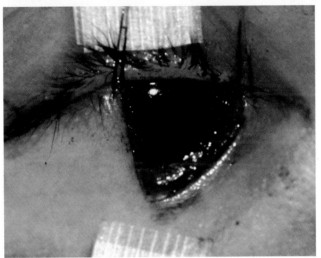

Figure 2.6

Irregular marginal defect converted to a full-thickness pentagonal defect with resection of the squared-off tarsal remnant, followed by excision of stepped-down triangles of skin, orbicularis, and septum/retractors/conjunctiva.

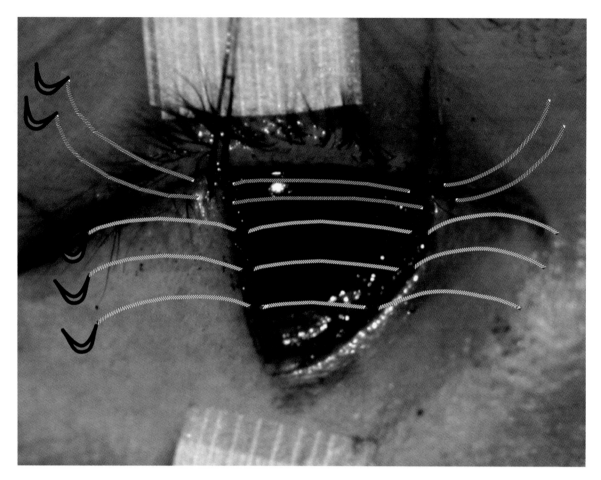

Figure 2.7

The direct approximation of a pentagonal defect follows the principles used in the repair of a full-thickness eyelid laceration: alignment with sutures through the gray line and the ciliary line (shown as blue/black sutures; 6-0 black silk preferred), and tension-bearing closure with sutures through the tarsus and eyelid retractors (shown as white/black sutures; 6-0 polyglactin 910 preferred). A third marginal suture can be placed at the level of the Meibomian gland orifices, but should be avoided if postoperative corneal contact appears likely. Two or three buried 7-0 polyglactin 910 sutures in orbicularis muscle/subdermal tissue decrease tension across the skin wound. The latter is closed with running 7-0 nylon suture, which is also tied over the ends of the marginal silk sutures, left long to avoid corneal irritation (see Figs. 2.8 and 2.9).

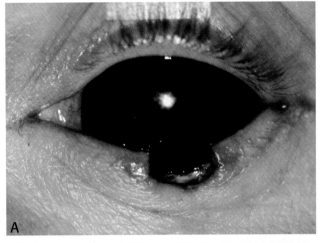

Figure 2.8

A. An irregular defect has been converted to a pentagon. **B.** A 6-0 black silk suture temporarily aligns the marginal edges. **C.** Retraction of skin with Steri-Strips exposes tarsal and retractor edges for closure with 6-0 polyglactin 910 sutures.

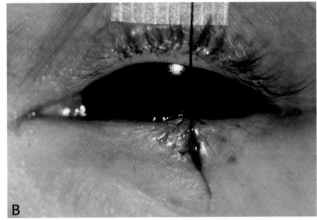

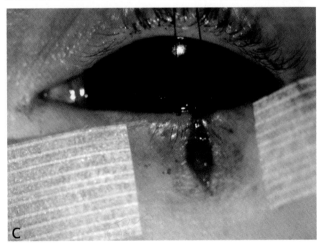

Figure 2.9

A. After closure of the posterior lamella, a second marginal silk suture is passed at the level of the cilia. **B.** The marginal sutures are tied, and buried 7-0 polyglactin 910 sutures are passed through orbicularis muscle/ subdermal tissue. **C.** The skin edges are closed with 7-0 nylon suture, which is tied over the long ends of the marginal silk sutures.

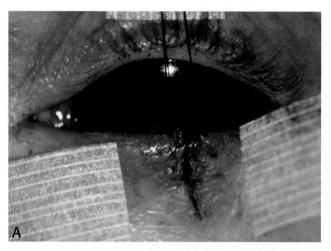

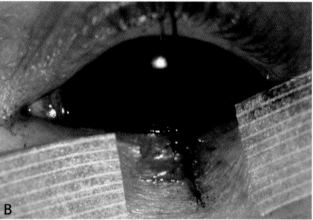

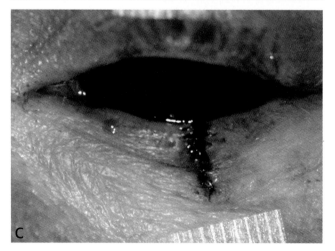

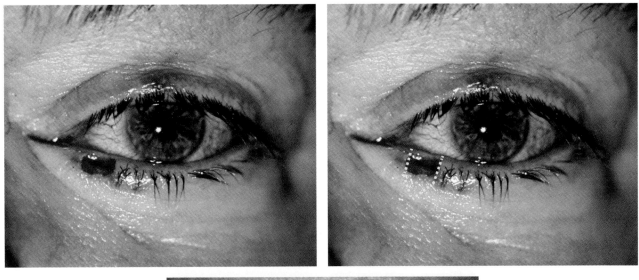

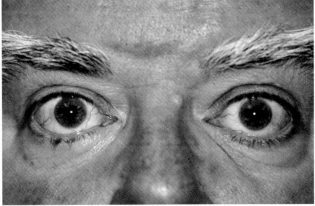

Figure 2.10

Small defect extending into superficial tarsus. Conversion to a full-thickness pentagonal defect and direct closure restore marginal continuity without an obvious lashless zone.

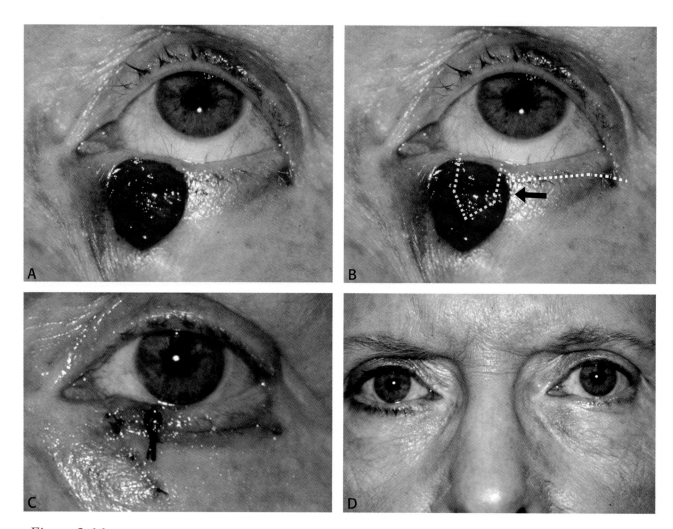

Figure 2.11

A. Because basal cell carcinomas arise in the anterior lamella, saucer-shaped Mohs defects generally involve more skin than tarsus. **B.** Full-thickness pentagonal excision and closure of the tarsal component restore marginal continuity, and the residual nonmarginal defect can be resurfaced with an advancement skin flap (see Chapter 3 for a discussion of skin flaps used in reconstruction of nonmarginal lower eyelid defects). **C.** Patient 1 week after surgery. **D.** Patient 1 year after surgery (makeup removed).

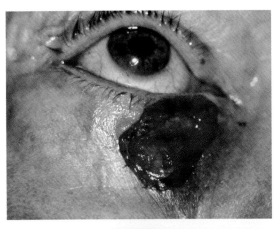
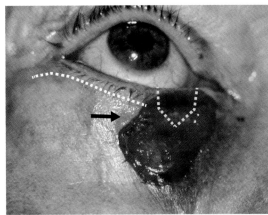
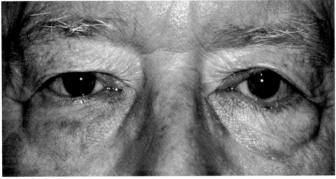

Figure 2.12

An 85-year-old man with a partial-thickness tarsal defect, moderate eyelid margin laxity, and taut, inelastic skin. Reconstruction included an 8-mm pentagonal resection/repair and an advancement skin flap dissected beyond the lateral canthus.

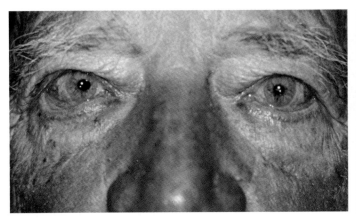
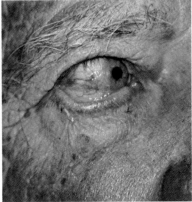

Figure 2.13

A 90-year-old man with bilateral ectropion (right greater than left) related to both horizontal laxity and vertical traction. The latter resulted from chronic dermatitis affecting both eyes, and from prior surgery for a basal cell carcinoma of the right lower eyelid—now recurrent (see Figs. 2.14 and 2.15).

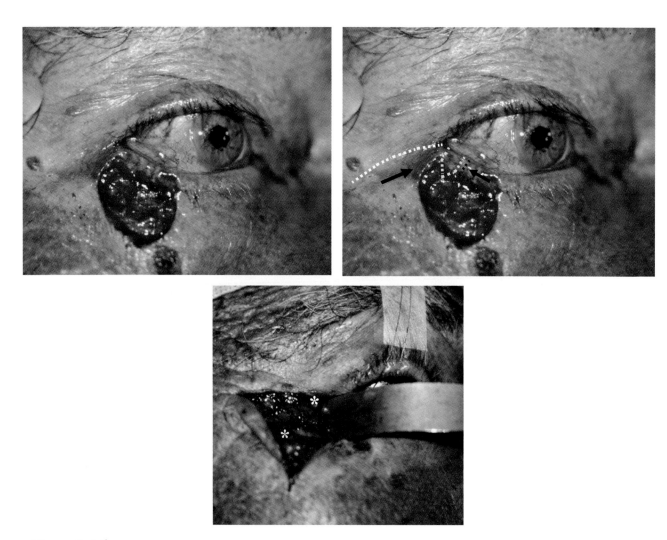

Figure 2.14

Following Mohs excision, the marginal defect and horizontal laxity were addressed with a small pentagonal excision (yellow lines) and a lateral tarsal strip procedure (blue lines; see Figs. 3.9–3.11). The remaining nonmarginal defect was resurfaced with an advancement flap anchored from its subcutaneous surface (yellow asterisk) to the periosteum of the lateral orbital rim (white asterisk). (See Chapter 3 for a discussion of anchored cheek flaps.)

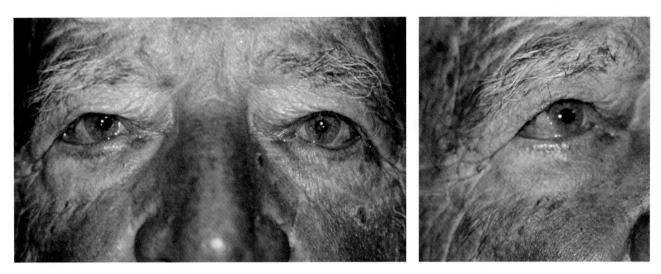

Figure 2.15

Patient depicted in Figures 2.13 and 2.14 1 year after right lower eyelid reconstruction.

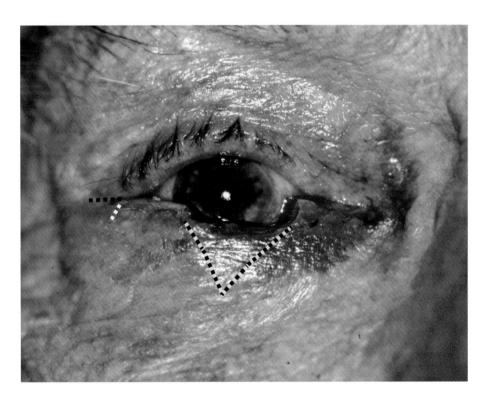

Figure 2.16

If defect width and marginal tension do not allow direct approximation, relaxation can be initiated with a small lateral canthal skin incision (black dotted line) and an *internal* cantholysis of the lower limb of the lateral canthal tendon (white dotted line). The pentagonal defect is then closed in standard fashion. The lateral canthal incision is not sutured (see Figs. 2.17 and 2.18).

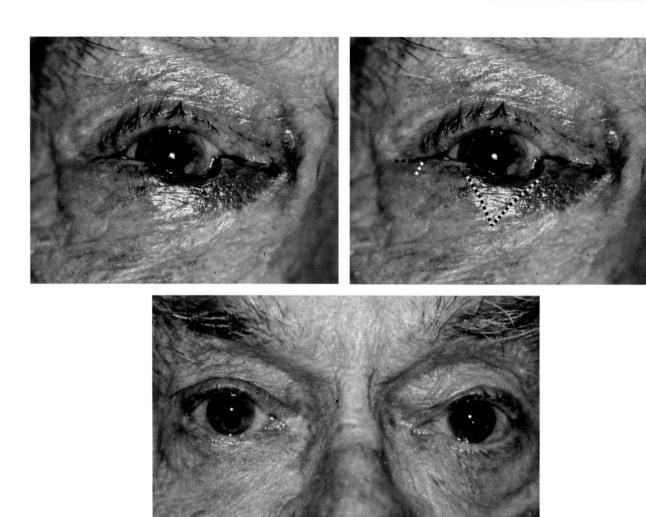

Figure 2.17

A 79-year-old man with a 1.5-cm marginal defect reconstructed with standard bilamellar reapproximation after a small lateral canthotomy/cantholysis. The patient 8 months after surgery.

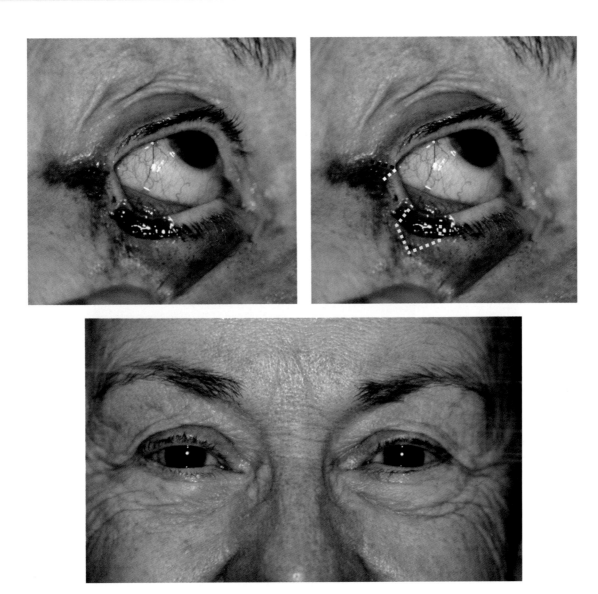

Figure 2.18

A 77-year-old woman with a 1.4-cm marginal defect repaired with direct approximation after lateral cantholysis. The patient 9 months after surgery.

Figure 2.19

The lateral canthal tendon and orbital septum are a connective tissue continuum that suspends and anchors the lateral tarsus. Internal cantholysis can be continued as internal release of the orbital septum (white dotted arrow) as far as the inferior orbital rim, titrating the degree of relaxation to that needed for marginal approximation (see Figs. 2.20 and 2.21).

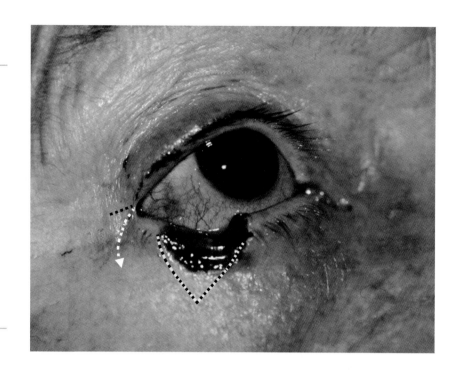

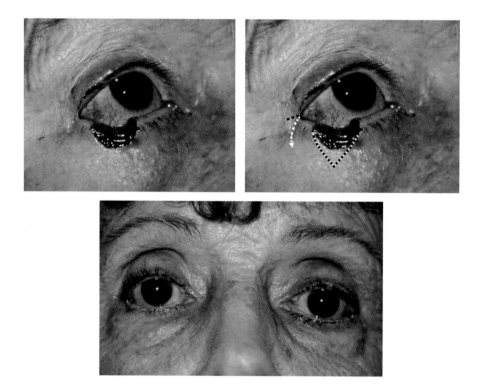

Figure 2.20

An 81-year-old woman with a 1.3-cm marginal defect, repaired with conversion to a pentagonal defect and direct approximation after inferior cantholysis and orbital septum release. The patient 6 months after surgery.

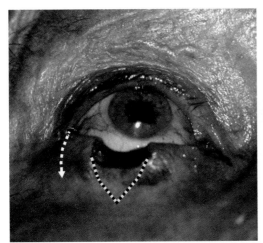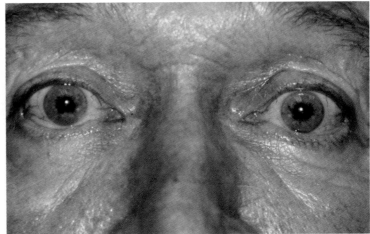

Figure 2.21

A 78-year-old man with a 1.3-cm marginal defect. Reconstruction involved pentagonal resection, internal cantholysis with partial orbital septum release (white dotted arrow), and standard bilamellar marginal repair. The patient 5 months after surgery, with slightly greater scleral show of the operated eye.

Figure 2.22

If defect width exceeds the capacity of lateral cantholysis plus septal release because of tension in the anterior lamella, additional tissue can be recruited by elevating a convexity-up, semicircular flap (black dotted line), as described by Tenzel[1] (see Figs. 2.23, 2.24, and 2.26–2.31).

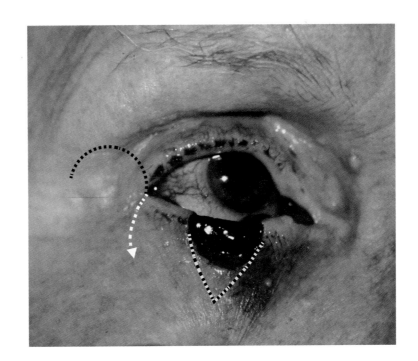

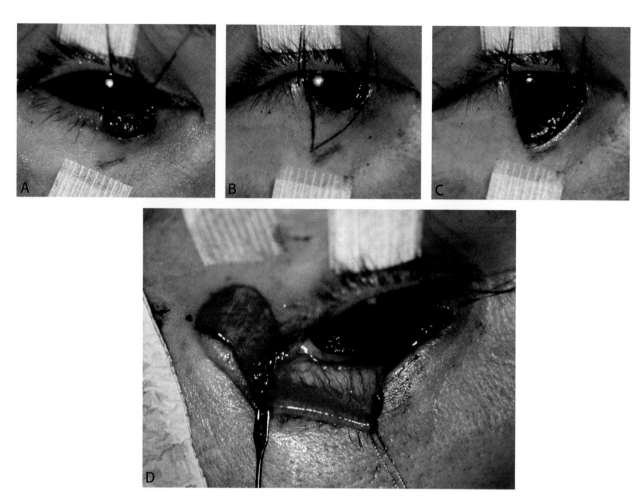

Figure 2.23

A–C. Final commitment to a semicircular rotation flap (rather than an eyelid-sharing procedure) is not necessary until the irregular tarsal defect is "squared off" and horizontal tension can be tested with traction sutures. The pentagonal resection is then completed.
D. The semicircular incision begins at the lateral canthus and ends over the lateral palpebral raphe, with a diameter of 12 to 15 mm. My preference is flap dissection at the subcutaneous level, rather than at the submuscular level as originally described. Cantholysis of the lower limb of the lateral canthal tendon and release of the orbital septum follow. The residual lateral eyelid is therefore mobilized as a full-thickness pedicle flap.

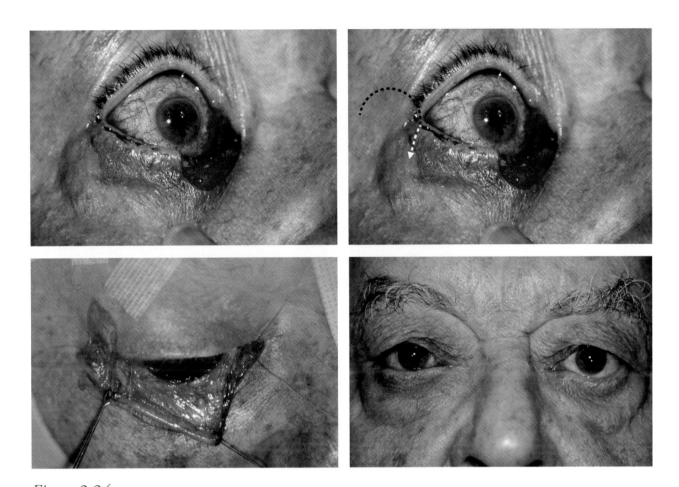

Figure 2.24

A 78-year-old man with a one-third to one-half lower eyelid defect extending into the lower canaliculus. Reconstruction included a semicircular flap, inferior cantholysis and septum release, bicanalicular nasolacrimal intubation (see Fig. 2.25), and anchoring to the medial canthal tendon. Closure of the semicircular flap includes resuspension to the intact superior limb of the lateral canthal tendon with a single buried 6-0 polyglactin 910 suture.

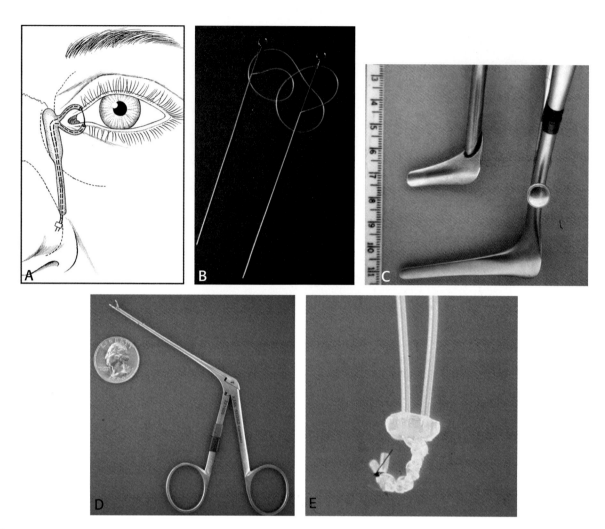

Figure 2.25

Canalicular stenting to maintain lacrimal outflow is included in the reconstruction of marginal eyelid defects that extend medial to the lacrimal puncta. Bicanalicular–nasal intubation allows the stents to be maintained for as long as several months without interfering with drainage. **A.** Schematic depiction of the lacrimal drainage system stented with silicone tubing. (Modified and reproduced with permission from Elsevier. Source: Harris GJ, Fuerste FH. Lacrimal intubation in the primary repair of midfacial fractures. Ophthalmology 1987;94:242–247.) Based on the technique originally described by Quickert and Dryden,[2] the method I favor uses the C-line intubation set (Medtronic Xomed, Inc., Jacksonville, FL) **(B)**. The sheathed probes are directly visualized in the inferior meatus with a fiberoptic headlight and a long, flat narrow-billed nasal speculum (**C**, lower instrument) inserted lateral to the inferior turbinate. The stylette/probe is removed, and the sheath and attached tubing are engaged and extracted with a micropituitary cup forceps **(D)**. The tubing is passed through a silicone button (Labtician Ophthalmics, Inc., Oakville, ON), which is trimmed to reduce its bulk, and the tubing is tied to itself with multiple knots and 6-0 nylon suture distal to the knots **(E)**. The stent is removed 3 months after surgery.

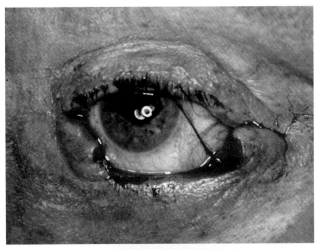
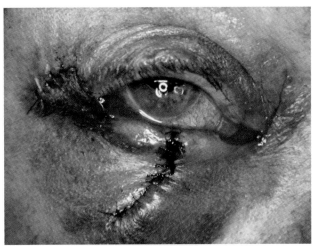
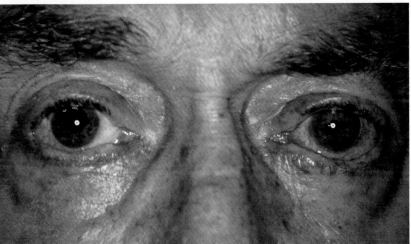

Figure 2.26

The sizes of defects amenable to semicircular flap reconstruction vary with residual tissue distensibility, but defects of at least one-half eyelid width can often be repaired in elderly patients. Considering the necessary relaxation of deep lateral canthal and orbital rim attachments, moderate tension should be the intraoperative end point if postoperative ectropion is to be avoided. The range of defects responsive to this technique is demonstrated in Figures 2.27 to 2.31.

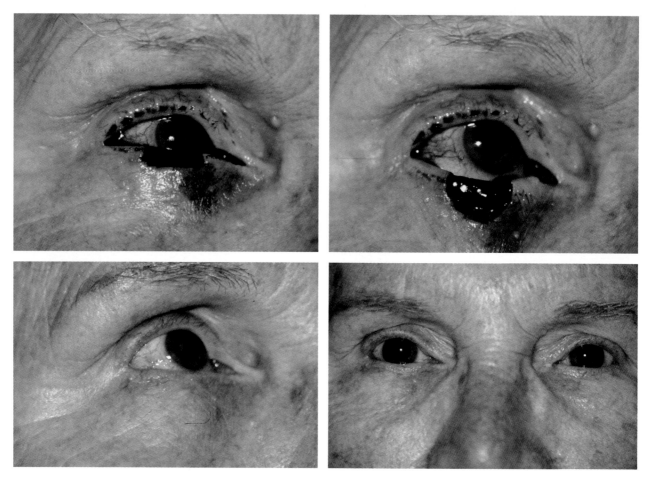

Figure 2.27

Semicircular flap reconstruction in a 79-year-old woman with a 1.1-cm right lower eyelid defect. Patient 5 months after surgery.

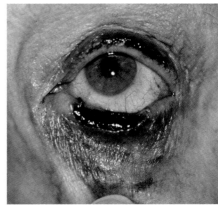
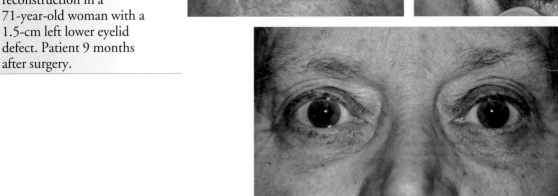
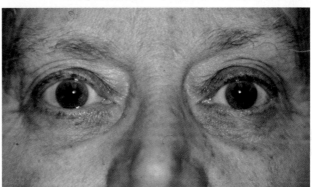

Figure 2.28

Semicircular flap reconstruction in a 71-year-old woman with a 1.5-cm left lower eyelid defect. Patient 9 months after surgery.

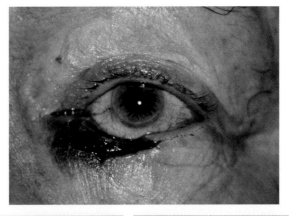

Figure 2.29

Semicircular flap reconstruction in a 72-year-old man with a 1.8-cm left lower eyelid defect extending to within 2 mm of the punctum. Patient 6 months after surgery. Note medial migration of isolated hair, but no canthal deformity.

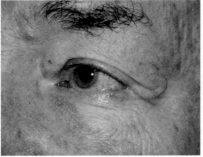
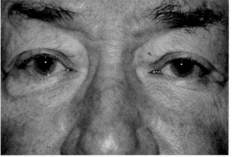

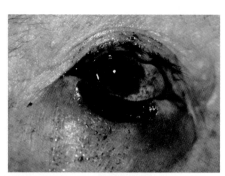

Figure 2.30

Semicircular flap reconstruction in an 86-year-old man with a 2.0-cm (one-half to two-thirds width) defect. Patient 3 months after surgery.

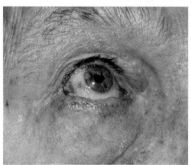

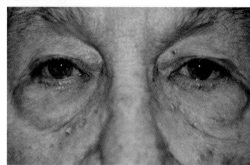

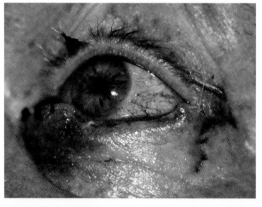

Figure 2.31

Semicircular flap reconstruction in a 48-year-old man with a 1.8-cm (one-half to two-thirds) defect of the left lower eyelid. Patient 1 year after surgery.

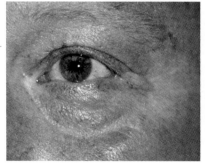

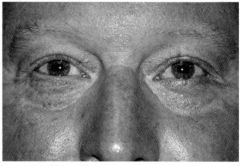

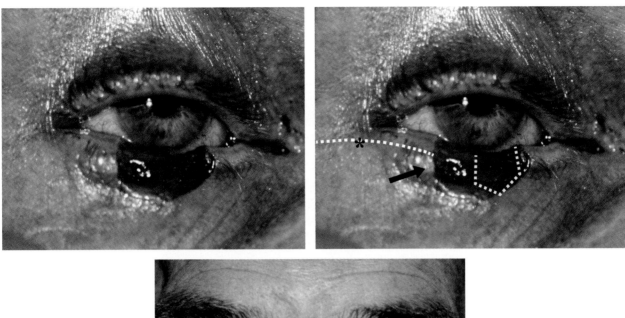

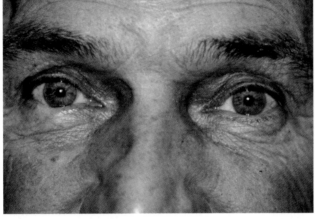

Figure 2.32

A 59-year-old man with a broad defect relative to eyelid tension, precluding repair with a semicircular flap. To narrow the lashless zone and avoid eyelid sharing, reconstruction included pentagonal resection/repair of the deeper medial half and an advancement skin flap anchored at the lateral orbital rim (asterisk) and raised to the margin (see Chapter 3 for a discussion of anchored advancement flaps). Patient 10 months after surgery.

Figure 2.33

If defect width does not allow edge approximation using the aforementioned techniques, an eyelid-sharing procedure is necessary. Options include a tarsoconjunctival flap resurfaced with a skin graft or flap, and a tarsal free graft resurfaced with a flap.

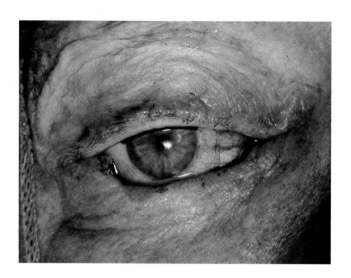

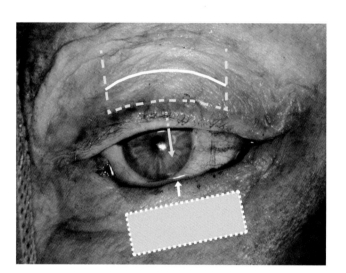

Figure 2.34

The classic Wendell Hughes[3] procedure combines a tarsoconjunctival transposition flap from the upper eyelid with a full-thickness skin graft. The upper eyelid is everted, and the height of the required tarsus is measured downward from the upper tarsal border (white solid line), maintaining at least 4 mm of marginal tarsus. The flap width is 2 mm less than the defect width, as measured with moderate tension on the defect edges. Flap dissection is performed between the tarsus and overlying levator aponeurosis to the upper tarsal border, and then between the conjunctiva and Mueller muscle. Dissection continues high enough into the upper fornix that the flap can be transposed without causing postoperative traction on the aponeurosis. The flap is sutured with 6-0 polyglactin 910 to the medial and lateral tarsal edges or canthal tendon remnants, and to the residual inferior eyelid retractors. In order of preference, and depending on its abundance, skin to surface the tarsoconjunctival flap is harvested from the ipsilateral or contralateral upper eyelid, from both upper eyelids, or from the postauricular region (see Figs. 2.35 and 2.36).

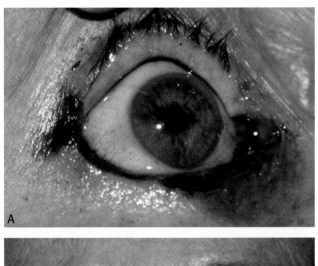

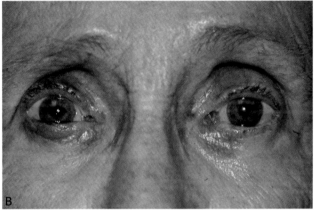

Figure 2.35

A. Defect of the entire right lower eyelid and lower canaliculus, repaired with bicanalicular nasolacrimal intubation, a full-width tarsoconjunctival flap, and a skin graft from the right upper eyelid. The medial 2 mm of the transposed flap was split longitudinally and was sutured posterior and anterior to the lacrimal stent with 6-0 and 7-0 polyglactin, respectively. The flap was separated 6 weeks later. **B.** Patient 3 months after primary repair, with some visibility of the graft. The disadvantage of palpebral fissure occlusion can be mitigated by opening a central window in the flap. Separation can also be accelerated to 2 to 3 weeks after primary repair, but longer attachment helps to counter downward traction as the wound bed fibroses.

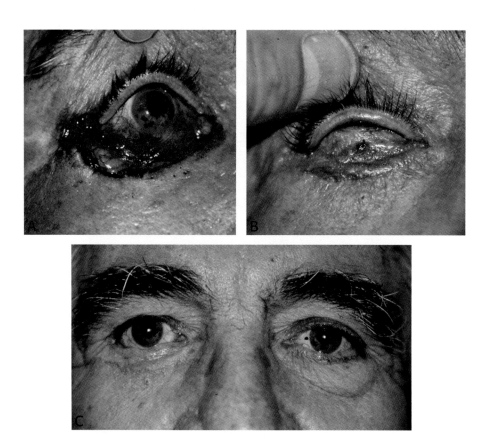

Figure 2.36

A. Defect involving the entire right lower eyelid, lateral canthus, and inferior canaliculus. Tissue loss extended posteriorly to the lower edge of the bulbar conjunctiva and anteriorly to the skin overlying the inferior orbital rim, with baring of orbital fat. Reconstruction included lacrimal intubation and a full-width Hughes flap covered with skin grafts from both upper eyelids. **B.** Patient 4 weeks after surgery. Because of anticipated fibrosis and contraction at the base of the defect, flap attachment and countertraction were maintained for 3 months. At the time of separation, with a grooved director behind the flap, an incision is made 1 to 2 mm above the desired final level of the margin. A 1- to 2-mm flap apron is retained in the upper eyelid, and its base is dissected and allowed to retract superiorly. **C.** Patient 4 months after primary repair, with a slightly irregular and erythematous eyelid margin.

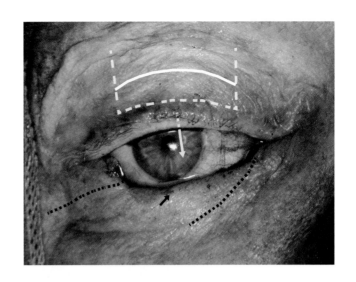

Figure 2.37

In cases with sufficiently lax and supple lower eyelid skin, the classic Hughes procedure can be modified with a horizontally directed skin flap as the anterior lamella replacement (see Fig. 2.38).

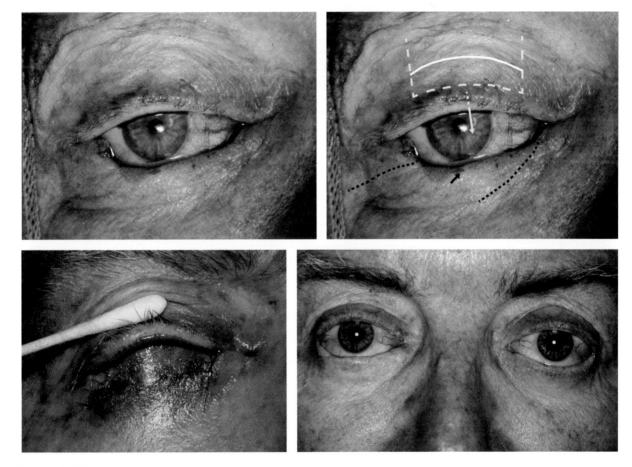

Figure 2.38

In my experience, the combination of flaps results in a more natural eyelid margin. Although the time of flap separation is not dictated by vascularization of an overlying graft, the attachment is maintained long enough to counter any downward traction observed during the early postoperative period.

Figure 2.39

The risk of late ectropion
may be reduced, and the
time of flap separation
accelerated, by resurfacing
the Hughes
tarsoconjunctival flap with
a laterally derived,
horizontally directed cheek
flap anchored to the
periosteum of the lateral
orbital rim (asterisk) (see
Fig. 2.40).

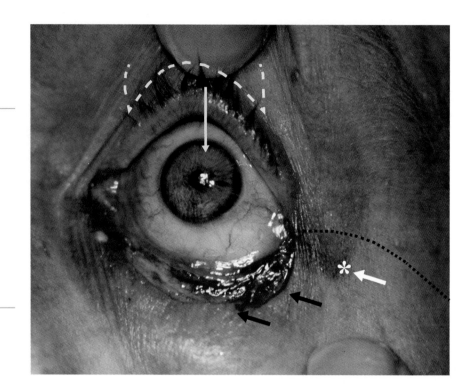

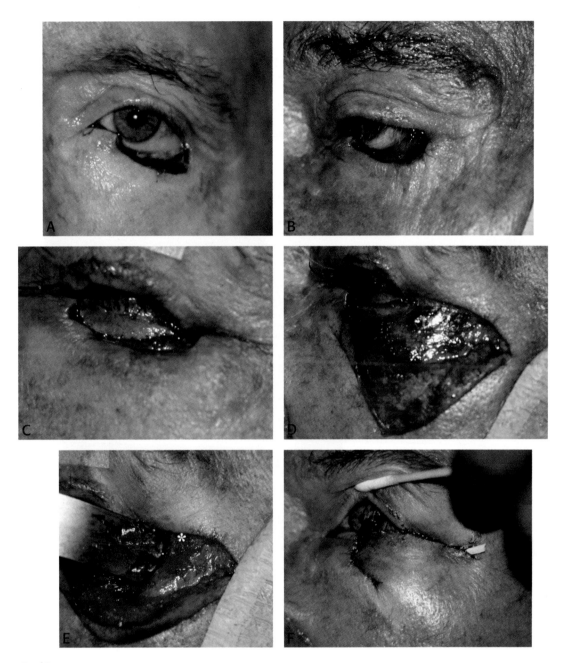

Figure 2.40

A, B. A broad defect, including the lower limb of the lateral canthal tendon. **C.** The tarsoconjunctival flap has been transposed and sutured to residual tarsus medially and to internal periosteum laterally. **D.** Using a relaxed skin tension line incision, a lower eyelid/ cheek flap has been raised. **E, F.** A retractor protects the orbital septum from a 4-0 polyglactin 910 suture to be passed through periosteum external to the orbital rim (asterisk), which will anchor the cheek flap. Because the anchor suture stretches the skin and also protects the eyelid from that traction, the relaxing incision and flap dissection need not be as extensive as those used for standard Mustardé cheek flaps.[4] (See Chapter 3 for a discussion of anchored lower eyelid/cheek flaps; see Figures 2.41 to 2.44 for results with combined Hughes and anchored flaps.)

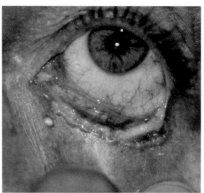 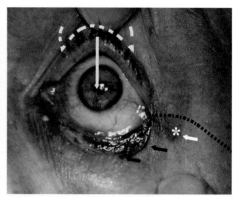

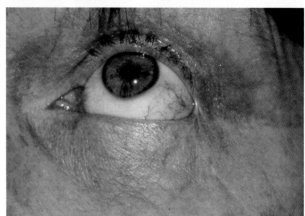

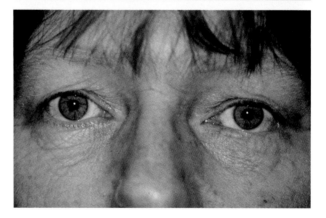

Figure 2.41

Combined Hughes and anchored cheek flaps. Extensive basal cell carcinoma had replaced the entire lower eyelid. Patient 1 year after surgery.

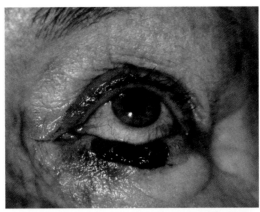

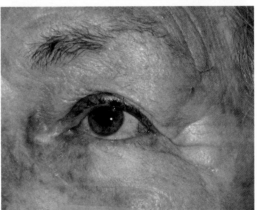

Figure 2.42

Combined Hughes and anchored cheek flaps used for repair of broad, shallow defect of left lower tarsus. Patient 6 months after surgery.

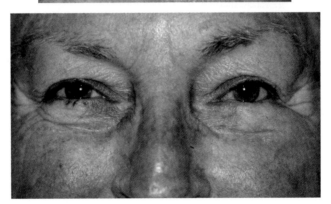

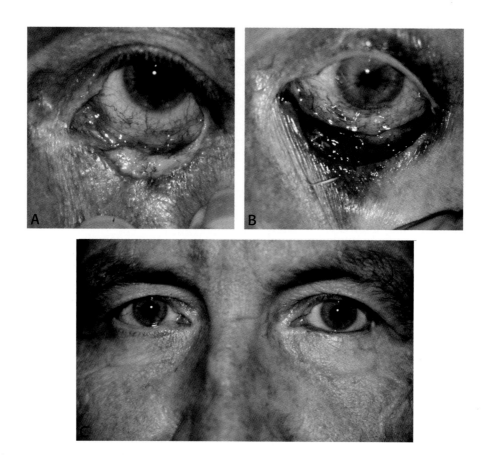

Figure 2.43

Combined Hughes and anchored cheek flaps. **A, B.** Extensive basal cell carcinoma and post-Mohs defect of the entire lower eyelid, including the lower canaliculus and conjunctiva of the medial lower fornix. The Hughes flap was extended to include conjunctiva of the medial upper fornix, and the medial edge of the tarsal portion was split for attachments both anterior and posterior to the lacrimal stent. **C.** Thirteen months after surgery, the eyelid position and lacrimal drainage are satisfactory, but vascularity at the junction of the tarsal and cheek flaps persists. Although not elected by the patient, this problem can respond to argon laser treatment.

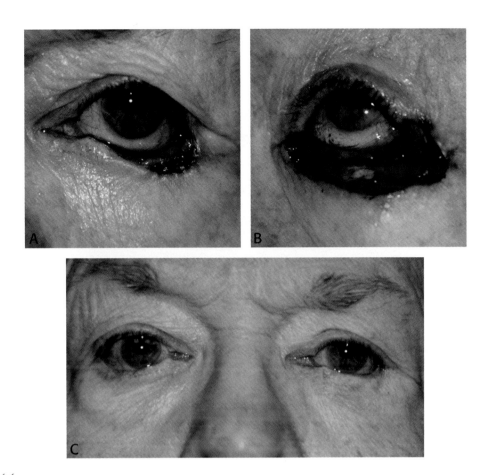

Figure 2.44

Combined Hughes and anchored temple/cheek flaps. **A, B.** Advanced basal cell carcinoma and post-Mohs defect involving the entire lower tarsus, part of the lower retractor complex, the lower limb of the lateral canthal tendon, and the skin of the lower eyelid, lateral canthus, and outer upper eyelid. A relaxing incision began at the superior pole of the defect within the upper eyelid and continued laterally to the hairline. After advancement and anchoring of the temple/cheek flap, a residual superomedial skin defect was resurfaced with a graft from the left upper eyelid (see Chapters 3 and 5 for a discussion of anchored cheek and temple flaps). **C.** The patient 1 year after primary repair. Bilateral, dermatitis-related lower eyelid retraction is slightly greater on the operated side.

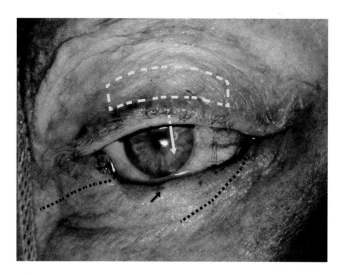

Figure 2.45

Another alternative to the classic Hughes procedure, described by Hawes,[5] replaces the posterior lamella with a free tarsal graft rather than a tarsoconjunctival flap. The tarsal graft is dissected in the manner of a Hughes flap, but it is amputated at the upper tarsal border. (Leaving a peripheral "frame" of tarsus can lead to upper eyelid distortion as the wound bed contracts.) An example of a free tarsal graft combined with a lower eyelid skin flap is shown in Figure 2.46.

Figure 2.46

A two-thirds lower eyelid defect repaired with a free tarsal graft from the ipsilateral upper eyelid and a horizontally oriented lower eyelid skin flap. By not occluding the palpebral fissure, the procedure benefits patients with better vision in the operated eye. It does not provide countertraction against gravitational and cicatricial forces, which may lead to ectropion or scleral show.

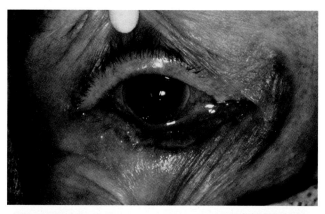

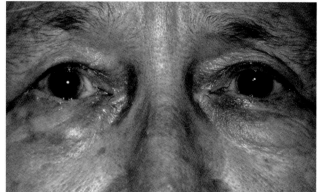

Figure 2.47

The risk of late ectropion when using a free tarsal graft may be reduced if the anterior lamella is replaced with a flap anchored to lateral orbital rim periosteum (asterisk). (See Chapter 3 for a discussion of anchored lower eyelid/cheek flaps. See Figures 2.48 and 2.49 for examples of combined free tarsal grafts and anchored flaps.)

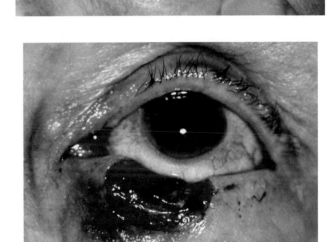

Figure 2.48

Broad, shallow tarsal defect. A tarsal graft from the opposing upper eyelid, sutured to the medial, lateral, and inferior defect edges, will be covered with a lower eyelid/cheek flap anchored to the lateral orbital rim.

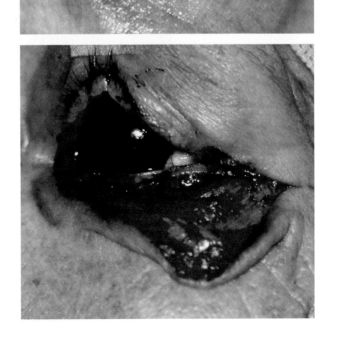

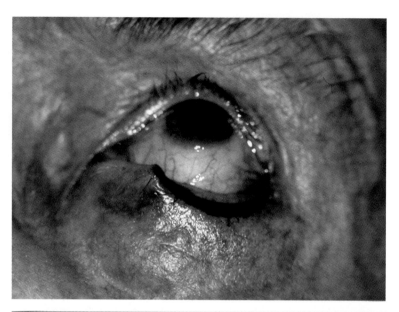

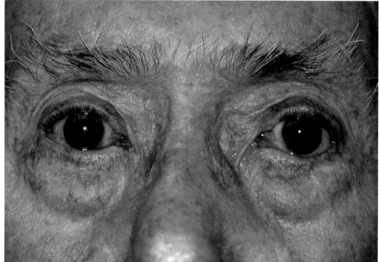

Figure 2.49

Defect involving two thirds of left lower eyelid, reconstructed with a free tarsal graft from the ipsilateral upper eyelid and an anchored lower eyelid/ cheek flap. Patient 8 months after surgery.

Although the less common lesions—sebaceous gland carcinoma and Merkel cell tumor—have predilections for the upper eyelids, basal cell carcinomas occur there far less frequently than on the lower eyelids. Reconstructive principles for the upper eyelids are generally similar to those for the lower eyelids, including the preferred approximation of defect edges before resorting to eyelid-sharing procedures. However, structural and functional differences between the upper and lower eyelids do have reconstructive implications.

That the eyelids and variably curved globe surface can move widely in relation to each other without losing apposition is permitted by compliance or elasticity of the eyelid tissues and their canthal attachments. As shown earlier, this "slack" is freely exploited in the reapproximation of lower eyelid defect edges. However, the considerably greater excursion of the upper eyelid over the corneal convexity can permit *over*exploitation in this regard. Although large lower eyelid defects can be closed with moderate tension that usually dissipates without deformity (e.g., Fig. 2.26), upper eyelid defects of similar size may be closed with less tension, but with permanent ptosis— particularly in patients with involutional weakness of the levator aponeurosis. In such cases, I try to minimize downward stretch of the aponeurosis by generously lysing lateral canthal and retinacular attachments. In addition, tarsal grafts or flaps are introduced earlier in the reconstructive "ladder."

Because tarsal heights are approximately 10 mm in the upper eyelid and 4 mm in the lower eyelid, and because at least 2 mm of lower tarsus should be retained for marginal stability, a large defect of the upper tarsus cannot be completely replaced by transfer from the lower eyelid. On the other hand, more abundant tarsus allows the upper eyelid to serve as its own graft or flap donor source in many cases.

Continuous contact and friction between the upper eyelid and cornea require that absorbable tarsal sutures either be nonbraided or do not extend through full-thickness tarsoconjunctiva. Posterior lamella replacement with palatal or nasal mucosa is generally avoided in all cases; use of these tissues in the upper eyelid is particularly likely to compromise the cornea.

Cases illustrating the reconstruction of upper eyelid margin defects are shown in Figures 2.50 to 2.69.

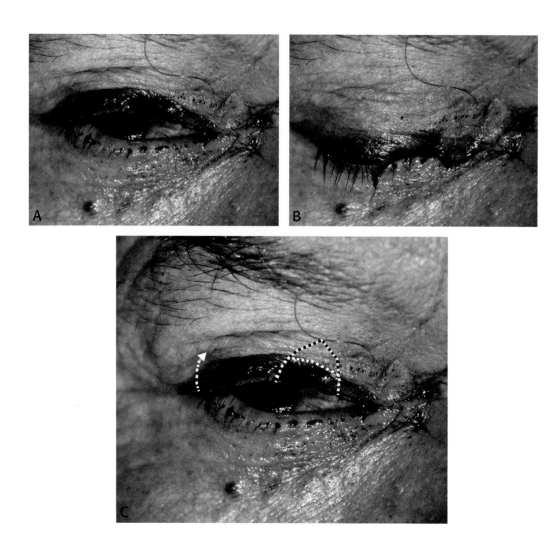

Figure 2.50

A, B. Upper eyelid defect involving a 10-mm marginal segment of tarsus. In elderly patients, the risk of postoperative ptosis with even mild horizontal tension requires generous relaxation of canthal attachments. **C.** Reconstruction included excision of the tarsal remnant (white dotted line); triangular excisions of skin, orbicularis, and retractors/conjunctiva (yellow line; see Figs. 2.5 and 2.19 for lower eyelid analogues); a small lateral canthotomy (black dotted line); and superior-limb cantholysis with partial release of the orbital septum and the lateral levator horn (white dotted arrow) (see Figure 2.51).

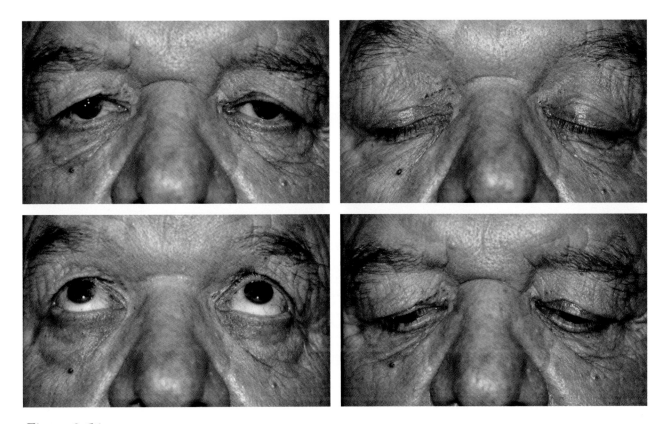

Figure 2.51

The patient 4 months after the right upper eyelid reconstruction depicted in Figure 2.50. The patient has involutional ptosis of the unoperated left eye.

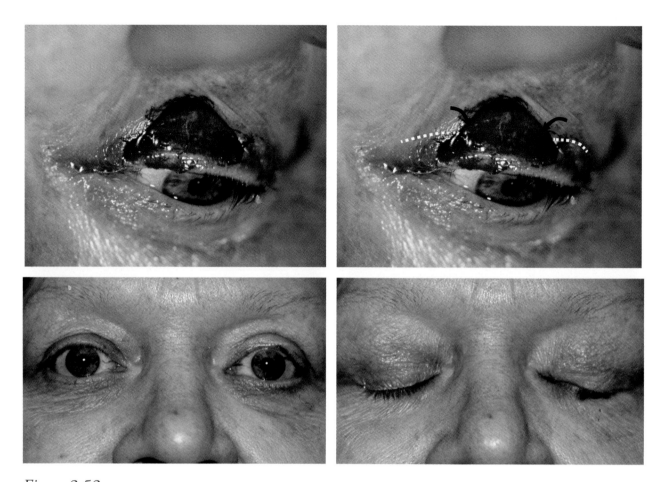

Figure 2.52

A 56-year-old patient with a broad defect through the cutaneous, but not the conjunctival, aspect of the eyelid margin—judged to be too broad to allow closure without a lashless segment, and too shallow for a tarsal graft or flap. Reconstruction involved medial and lateral eyelid crease incisions, with advancement of skin to the margin, and excision of a superior dog-ear. There is no exposure keratopathy.

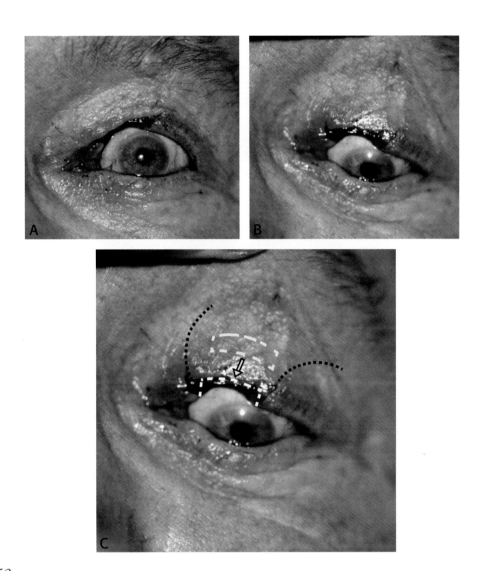

Figure 2.53

A, B. A left upper eyelid margin defect included an 11 × 3-mm tarsal segment. **C.** The tarsal defect was "squared off" (white dotted line) and a free tarsal graft (yellow dotted line) was harvested from the superior aspect of the same tarsus. The graft was secured with 6-0 polydioxanone monofilament suture with anterior knots, and was surfaced with a skin flap (black dotted lines) sutured at the eyelid margin with running 7-0 nylon (see Fig. 2.54).

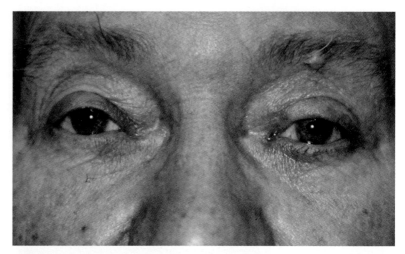

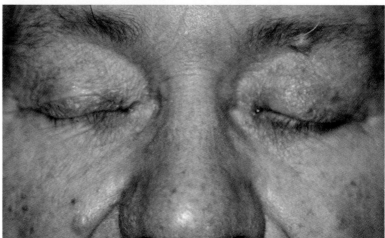

Figure 2.54

The patient 4 months after the left upper eyelid reconstruction depicted in Figure 2.53.

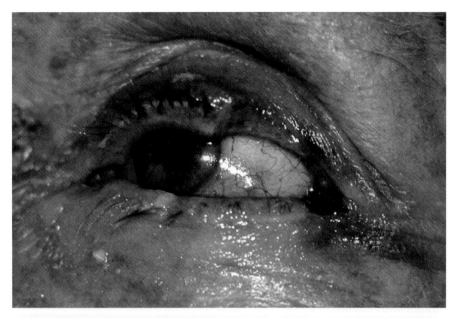

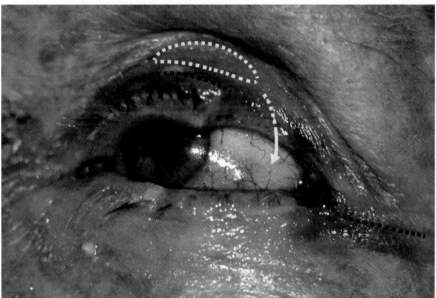

Figure 2.55

A 12 × 2.5-mm defect of tarsus and levator aponeurosis, with a larger anterior lamellar deficit. A similar-size graft from the upper tarsal border was sutured to residual tarsus medially with two 6-0 chromic catgut sutures, to the remnant of canthal tendon laterally with two 6-0 polyglactin 910 sutures, and to residual tarsus and levator aponeurosis superiorly with running 6-0 plain catgut suture. Using incisions in the natural upper eyelid crease and a crow's-foot, a large skin flap was elevated. The lateral aspect, anchored to periosteum of the orbital rim with a buried 5-0 polyglactin 910 suture, was advanced to cover the tarsal graft partially. The medial aspect was advanced and sutured to the new eyelid margin with running 7-0 nylon. A small triangle of redundant skin was excised superiorly (see Fig. 2.56).

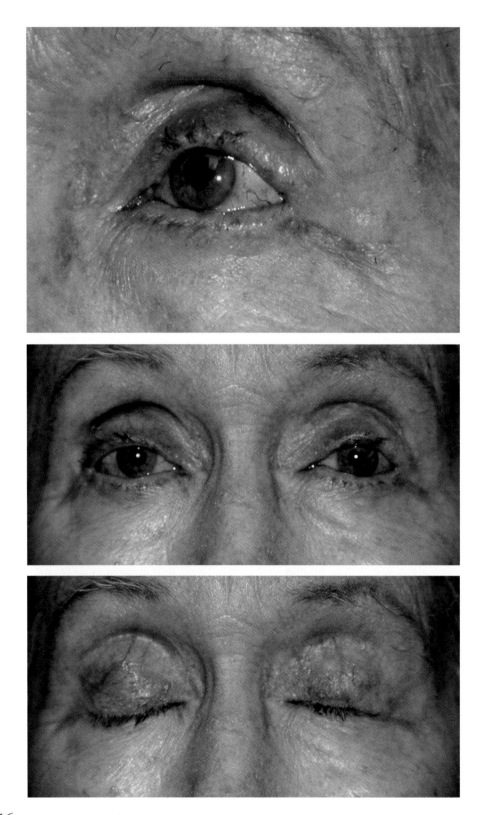

Figure 2.56

The patient 1 year after the left upper eyelid reconstruction shown in Figure 2.55.

Figure 2.57

If there is concern about revascularization of a free tarsal graft, a tarsoconjunctival flap can be used for posterior lamellar replacement. **A.** A defect involving a 20 × 8-mm anterior lamellar deficit and an 11 × 3-mm tarsal segment in a diabetic patient. **B.** A Hughes-type flap was transposed to the eyelid margin and sutured to the squared-off tarsal edges with 7-0 chromic catgut. Conjunctiva of the "leap-frogged" tarsal bridge was abraded with a scalpel. Medial eyelid crease and lateral crow's-foot incisions were used to develop a skin flap, which was anchored laterally at the orbital rim with a buried 5-0 polyglactin 910 suture and fixed to the new tarsal margin with running 7-0 nylon suture (see Fig. 2.58).

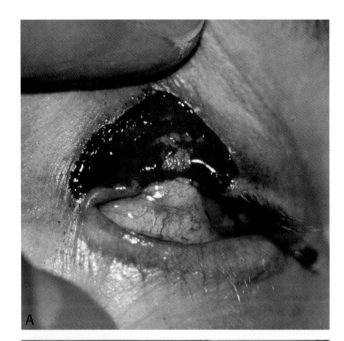

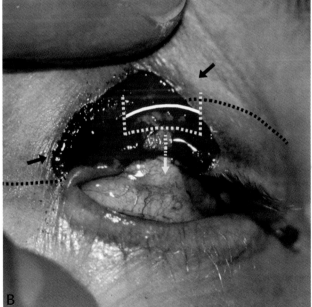

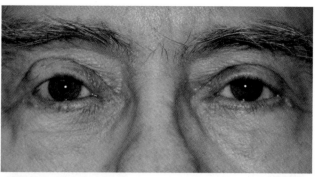

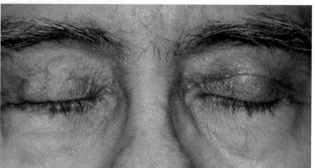

Figure 2.58

The patient 10 months after reconstruction of the right upper eyelid depicted in Figure 2.57.

Figure 2.59

A. A marginal defect extending to but not involving the right upper punctum. **B.** Reconstruction with a tarsoconjunctival flap transposed to the margin and resurfaced with a skin flap (see Fig. 2.60).

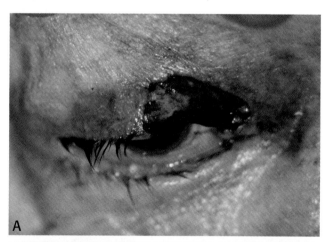

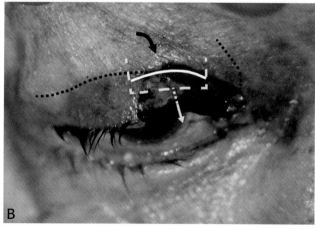

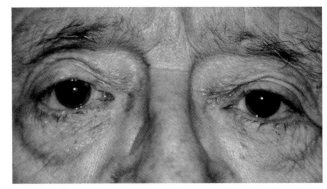

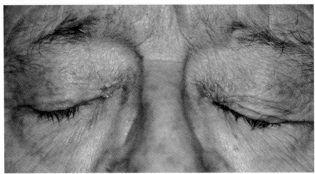

Figure 2.60

The patient 1 year after the reconstruction depicted in Figure 2.59.

Figure 2.61

A. A defect involving a 15 × 4-mm segment of tarsus, repaired with a superolaterally derived tarsoconjunctival flap and advancement skin flaps in the manner depicted in Figures 2.57 and 2.59.
B. The patient 6 months after surgery, showing the conjunctival aspect of the reconstructed right upper eyelid (see Fig. 2.62).

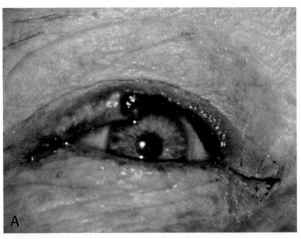

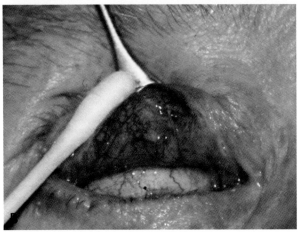

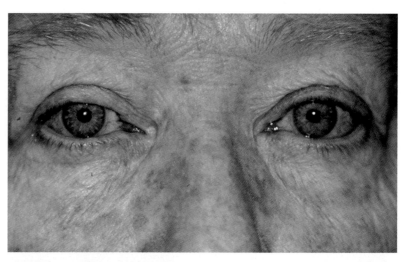

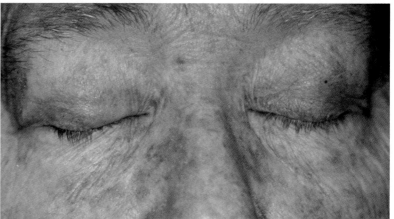

Figure 2.62

The patient shown in Figure 2.61, 6 months after right upper eyelid reconstruction.

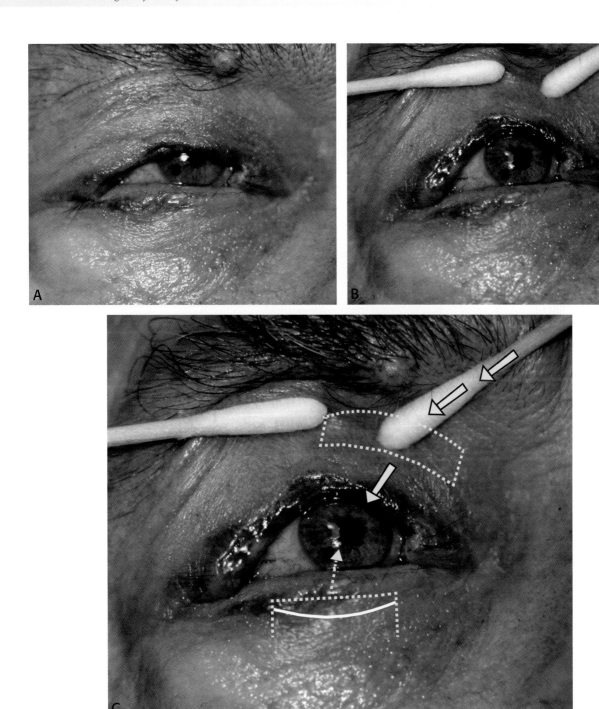

Figure 2.63

A 76-year-old man referred with a right upper eyelid lesion of 6 months' duration. Biopsy revealed Merkel cell tumor. **A, B.** Mohs resection included the central half of the tarsus, to within 2 to 3 mm of its upper border. **C.** Reconstruction involved a reverse Hughes flap from the lower eyelid and a free tarsal graft from the left (contralateral) upper eyelid (see Fig. 2.64).

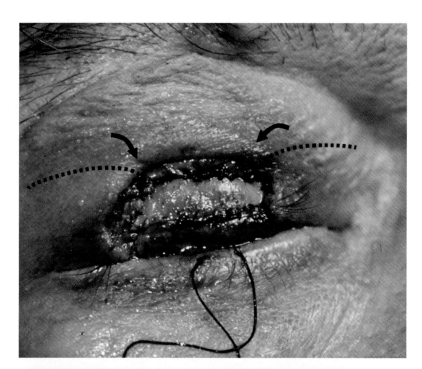

Figure 2.64

After posterior lamellar
components were
positioned and sutured
with 7-0 chromic catgut, a
myocutaneous flap (in
anticipation of
postoperative irradiation)
was advanced to the new
margin. Systemic workup
was negative. Flaps were
divided at 7 weeks. The
patient was tumor free
6 years later when he died
from unrelated causes.

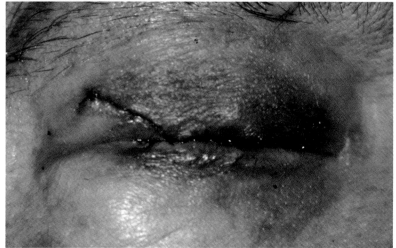

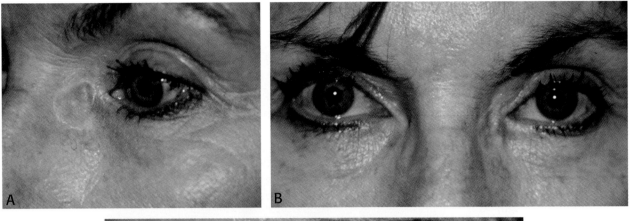

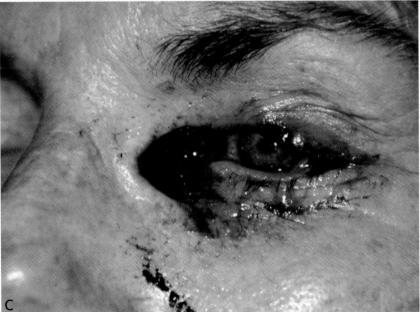

Figure 2.65

A, B. A basal cell carcinoma, first diagnosed 10 years earlier, had been resected on three occasions at another institution. Prior reconstruction included a postauricular skin graft. Biopsy revealed recurrent tumor. **C.** After Mohs resection, the defect measured 3.3 × 1.7 cm and involved the left medial canthus, including the upper and lower canaliculi, the medial half of the upper eyelid, including the full height of tarsus in that area, and the medial lower eyelid.

Figure 2.66

Reconstruction included a tarsoconjunctival flap advanced from the superior aspect of residual tarsus to the medial eyelid margin and the posterior lacrimal crest, where it was anchored with 4-0 polyglactin 910 suture. A lateral canthotomy, internal cantholysis, and retinaculum release (white dotted arrow) allowed mobilization. The medial aspect of the lower tarsus was also sutured to the posterior lacrimal crest (see Figs. 2.67–2.69).

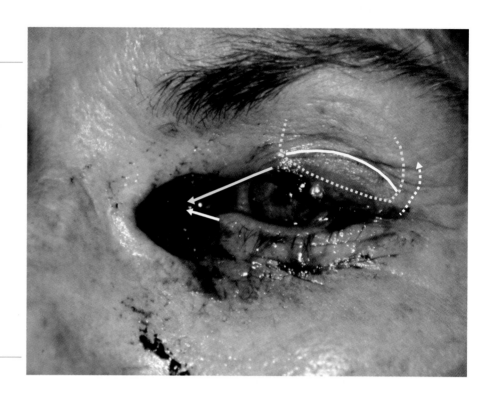

Figure 2.67

The tarsoconjunctival flap and the lower eyelid have been anchored to the posterior lacrimal crest.

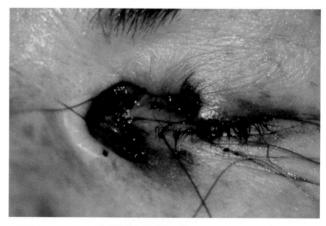

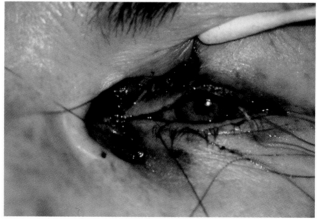

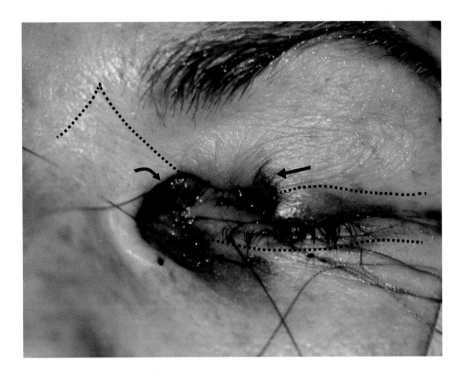

Figure 2.68

Reconstruction of the medial canthal and anterior lamellar eyelid defects was accomplished with glabellar, upper eyelid, and lower eyelid skin flaps, each anchored independently to the anterior limb of the medial canthal tendon. (See Chapter 4 for a discussion of multiple aesthetic unit flap reconstruction of medial canthal defects.)

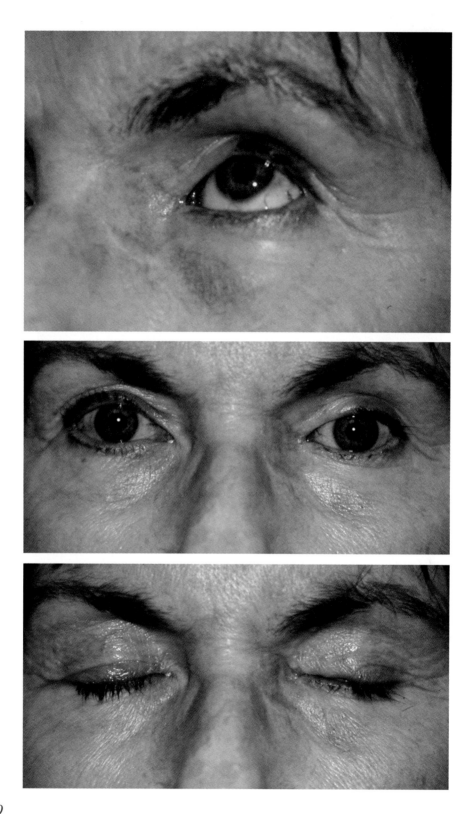

Figure 2.69

The patient 7 months after the surgery depicted in Figures 2.66 to 2.68. A conjunctivodacryocystorhinostomy with placement of a Lester Jones Pyrex tube was performed 5 months later.

Tissue-Loss Trauma

Marginal eyelid defects may also result from accidental or intentional trauma. (True tissue-loss should be distinguished from the considerable wound distraction that results from contraction of the transected tarsoligamentous sling and orbicularis muscle fibers toward their canthal insertions.) Compared with defects after Mohs surgery, traumatic defects are generally more irregular, and residual tissue may be crushed, sheared, or shredded; wounds may contain foreign debris and/or bacterial contaminants; and there may be associated injuries of the globe, orbital bones and soft tissues, or extraorbital structures. These factors often reduce the options for primary reconstruction from the full range available in the more controlled post-Mohs setting. For example, defects caused by animal or human bites, or by grossly contaminated industrial or farm implements, have high risks of infection. Those caused by high-speed impact or avulsion may be complicated by massive edema or hematoma. Because there is generally only one opportunity for the successful transposition of adjacent, opposing, or contralateral eyelid tissue, it is preferable to aim for globe protection during the primary repair, and to reserve complicated flaps for elective, secondary reconstruction.

Because of these many variables, a formulaic approach to post-trauma reconstruction is less applicable than in post-Mohs repair, but the same basic principles can be used with some improvisation. A few examples demonstrate concerns specific to traumatic tissue-loss (Figs. 2.70–2.80).

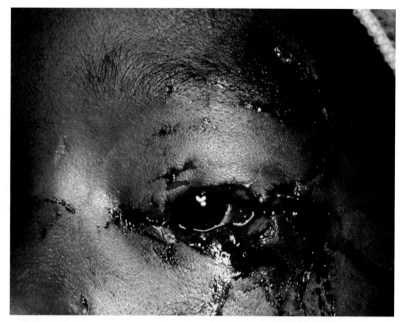

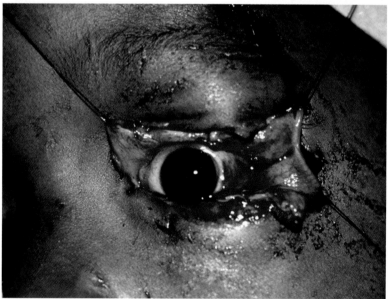

Figure 2.70

Dog-bite injury resulting in loss of the central half of the upper eyelid and the medial half of the lower eyelid, including the proximal canaliculus; laceration of the upper canaliculus; and traumatic disinsertion of the lateral canthal tendon. Management included intravenous antibiotics, pressure irrigation with saline (30-mL syringe, 30-gauge needle), and bicanalicular nasolacrimal intubation. The lateral canthus was divided horizontally to allow medial advancement of the upper and lower eyelid remnants. Mobilization required release of the orbital septum from the lateral orbital rim. The levator aponeurosis was dissected within the superior aspect of the wound and, after reapproximation of the eyelid margin, was sutured to the medially transposed upper tarsus (see Fig. 2.71).

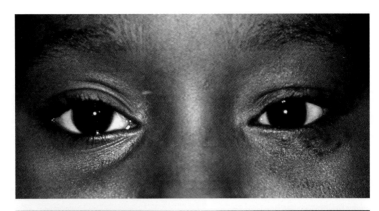

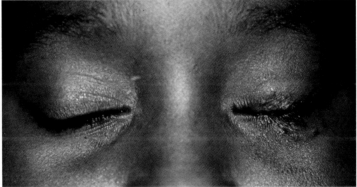

Figure 2.71

Late results after the primary repair described in Figure 2.70. Additional reconstruction was not elected.

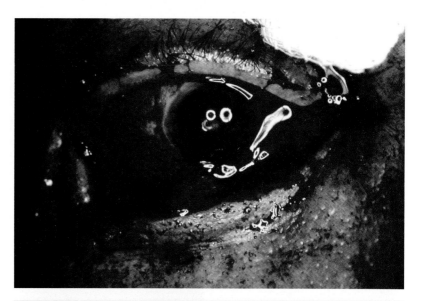

Figure 2.72

Avulsion of the entire right lower eyelid, except for a thin strip of lateral eyelid margin. The injury had been sustained in an industrial accident 4 hours before presentation to our institution. Coworkers at the 1-hour distant work site were contacted and asked to search for the missing tissue, and to transport it in ice (see Figs. 2.73 and 2.74).

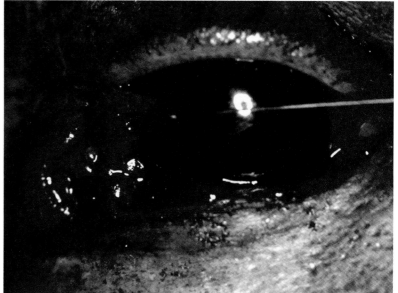

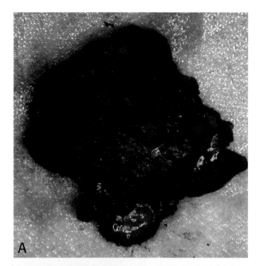

Figure 2.73

A. Missing tissue, upon delivery. **B, C.** Anterior and posterior aspects, respectively, of full-thickness eyelid (above) and "apron" of skin and muscle (below), after extensive cleansing.

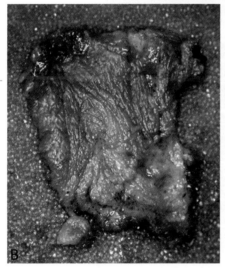

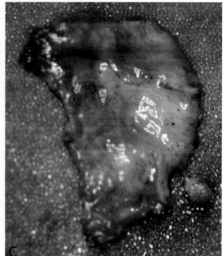

Figure 2.74

A. Immediately after replantation of the avulsed eyelid, the patient received the first of 12 hyperbaric oxygen treatments (to counter tissue hypoxia in the free graft by transdermal diffusion and to boost oxygen tension in the perfused recipient bed, thereby increasing the oxygen gradient and promoting capillary ingrowth). **B.** Patient at late follow-up. The more critical posterior lamella fully survived the primary repair; the anterior lamella has been augmented with a full-thickness skin graft. No additional reconstruction was needed.

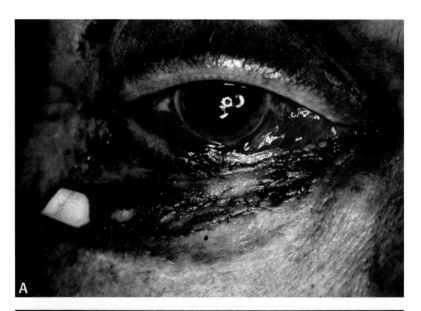

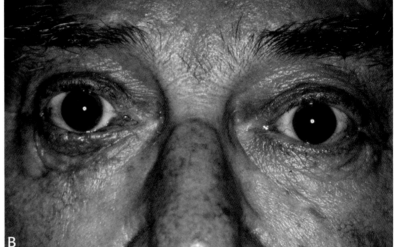

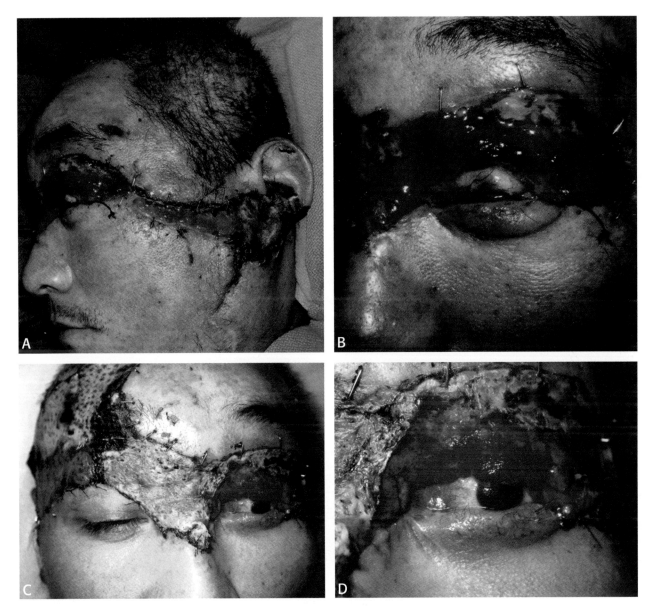

Figure 2.75

A, B A 38-year-old man had sustained a degloving injury involving his entire scalp, both eyebrows, left upper eyelid, and left ear when his hair became entangled in sawmill machinery 3 weeks earlier. The amputated tissues had been successfully replanted with meticulous microvascular anastomoses. Subsequent application of a halo fixation device caused compression of vessels and led to marginal necrosis and retraction. Tissue loss included the entire left upper eyelid. Split-thickness skin grafts were subsequently applied to bare and granulating areas; the left globe was protected with Frost sutures. (Photographs courtesy of James Sanger, MD.) **C, D.** Patient on presentation to the oculoplastic service. A shelf of exuberant, but unusable, granulation tissue now projected from muscle remnants on the orbital rim. Behind this, ragged edges of orbital septum, fat, levator muscle, and fornical conjunctiva were fused and contracted. The lower eyelid was intact (see Figs. 2.76–2.80).

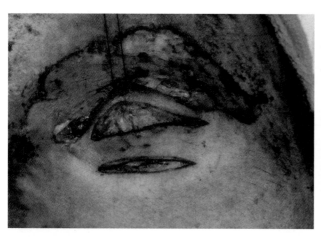
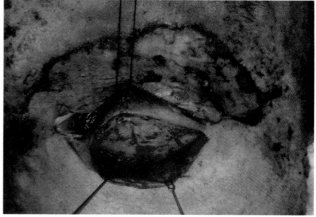

Figure 2.76

First-stage construction of a composite pedicle flap (additional split-thickness skin grafts had previously been applied to granulation tissue over the orbital rims). Roughly parallel relaxed skin tension line incisions (12 mm apart centrally) were made through lower eyelid preseptal skin and orbicularis muscle. The muscularis was undermined and the wounds were then closed. The flap was delayed to induce ischemia and increase collateral circulation.

Figure 2.77

A, B. One week after first-stage construction of a composite pedicle flap, with planning for second-stage flap lengthening and delay. (Lateral extension of the flap was limited by a previously dissected cheek flap used for other defects.) **C.** Patient immediately after flap extension, undermining, and resuturing. "Tarsorrhaphy" sutures were placed for corneal protection. One and 2 weeks later, the lateral edge ("third side") of the pedicle was partially transected and resutured to further delay the flap.

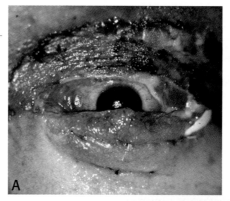
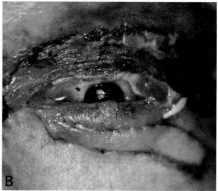
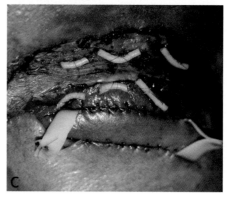

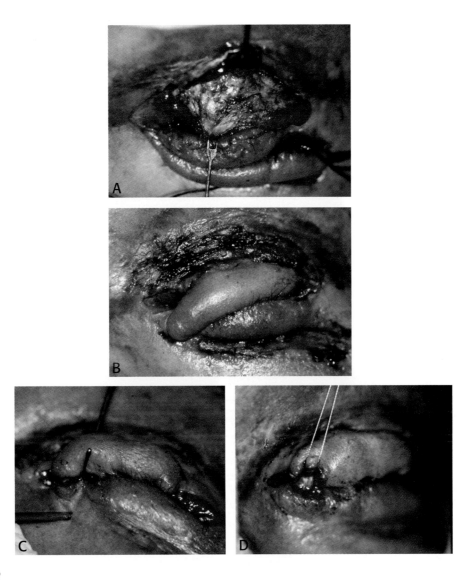

Figure 2.78

A. Twenty-six days after initial flap preparation. The flap was incised at its superior and inferior borders, and was undermined. Before the residual lateral pedicle was released, it was ligated to confirm capillary refill from the medial pedicle. The levator muscle was dissected from surrounding subbrow tissues, and the prolapsed lacrimal gland was separated from adhesions to the orbital rim. A split-thickness mucous membrane graft harvested from the buccal gutter was sutured to the posterior aspect of the flap. The transposed pedicle flap was sutured to levator muscle and infrabrow skin grafts superiorly, and to the deepithelialized lower eyelid margin inferiorly. The lower eyelid donor site was resurfaced with a full-thickness supraclavicular skin graft. **B.** Ten days after the transfer described in **(A)**. **C, D.** Staged division of the medial pedicle began 3 months after the transfer, and was completed 3 months later.

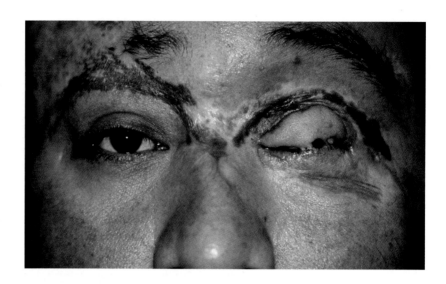

Figure 2.79

Patient 3 months after
final division and
transposition of the medial
pedicle to recipient skin
and conjunctiva of the
medial canthus. Pillar
tarsorrhaphies remain
intact.

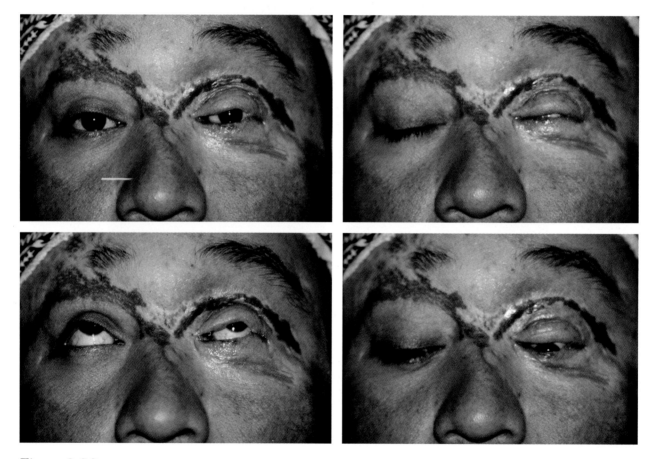

Figure 2.80

Patient 8 months after flap transposition, with interval release of tarsorrhaphies, lateral
canthal revision, and conservative trimming and debulking of the flap. In the absence of
upper eyelid orbicularis muscle (protractor) innervation, the patient's mechanical ptosis has
not been fully corrected. There is mild lagophthalmos, but no exposure keratopathy, and
vision remains normal.

References

1. Tenzel RR. Reconstruction of the central one half of an eyelid. Arch Ophthalmol 1975;93:125–126.
2. Quickert MH, Dryden RM. Probes for intubation in lacrimal drainage. Trans Am Acad Ophthalmol Otolaryngol 1970;74:431–433.
3. Hughes WL. A new method for rebuilding a lower lid. Arch Ophthalmol 1937;17:1008–1017.
4. Mustardé JC. Repair and Reconstruction in the Orbital Region. 2nd Ed. Edinburgh: Churchill Livingstone, 1980:52–57.
5. Hawes MJ. Free autogenous grafts in eyelid tarsoconjunctival reconstruction. Ophthalmic Surg 1987;18:37–41.

3

Nonmarginal Defects of the Lower Eyelid, Cheek, and Lateral Canthal Region

*M*any periocular tumors do not involve the eyelid margins directly, but their surgical resection and reconstructive outcomes can affect eyelid position. Nonmarginal defects of the mobile lower eyelid and lateral canthus are particularly vulnerable to gravity and downward traction (Fig. 3.1).

Skin grafts directly over healthy orbicularis muscle may succeed in the reconstruction of lower eyelid defects (Fig. 3.2). Mohs defects, however, often extend beyond the orbital perimeter, where wound beds are fatty and can be heavily cauterized during tumor resection. Several weeks after resurfacing, wound bed contraction can cause overlying skin grafts to shrink passively. In the periocular region, this generalized, nondirected contraction occurs at the expense of the mobile eyelid margin and lateral canthus (Fig. 3.3). Tarsorrhaphies can provide countertraction, but are impractical for the 6- to 8-week period needed. In addition, defects after Mohs resection may be deep, and because skin grafts must be thin to become vascularized, the resurfaced areas may be depressed.

With these concerns, local flaps are favored over grafts for reconstruction in this sector. Color and thickness matches are superior, and flap traction can be directed horizontally to offset the generalized bed shrinkage. Flaps tailored to follow the relaxed skin tension lines (RSTL)[1] (Fig. 3.4) usually blend better than flaps that conform to fixed geometric shapes. Adjunctive tightening of the lower eyelid margin—even if the defect does not extend to the margin—helps to stabilize it. Perhaps most important, anchoring flaps to deep, fixed tissue protects the eyelid margin from flap traction.[2] Anchored flaps are used for defects that extend to the medial or lateral orbital rims and for those that require flap dissection over the lateral rim.

For reconstruction after Mohs resection, we strive for same-day repair. If logistics require next-day reconstruction, an ophthalmic antibiotic ointment (e.g., erythromycin) and sterile eye pads are applied and maintained overnight, and an oral antibiotic (e.g., cephalexin) is prescribed. (Details of

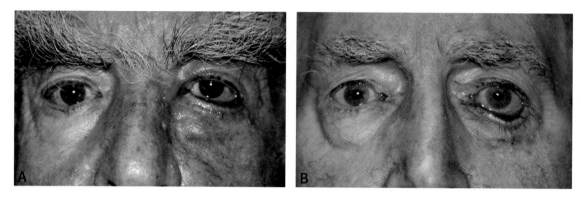

Figure 3.1

Two patients referred for ectropion repair after nonmarginal tumor-free defects had been reconstructed with a cheek flap (**A**) and a skin graft (**B**).

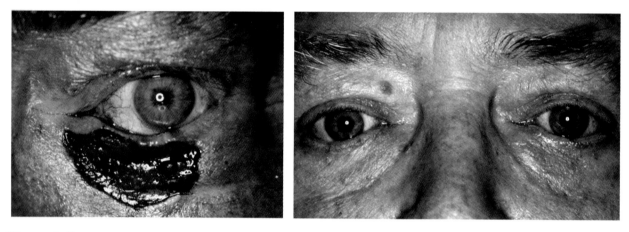

Figure 3.2

Skin from both upper eyelids was grafted directly to a lower eyelid bed of orbicularis muscle, without postoperative distortion.

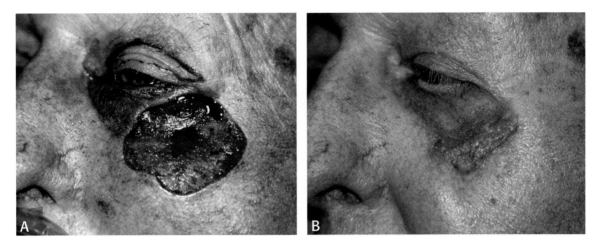

Figure 3.3

A. Post-Mohs defect of the lower eyelid and cheek, with a bed of exposed fat. Same-day resurfacing was performed with appropriate-size grafts (bilateral upper eyelid skin superiorly, thicker postauricular skin inferiorly). **B.** Six weeks later, fibrosis in the wound bed has caused passive contraction of the grafts. There is inferolateral eyelid and canthal traction, and a depressed, corrugated appearance.

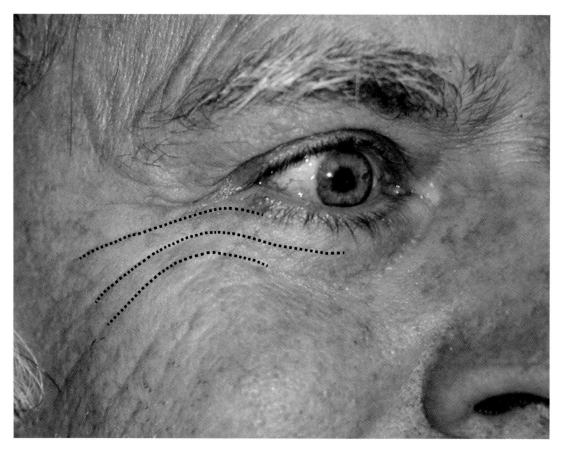

Figure 3.4

In the lower eyelid–cheek–lateral canthal sector, placement of relaxing incisions in natural creases and RSTL allows flap traction to be directed horizontally and minimizes incisional scarring.

the operative protocol are provided in Chapter 6.) With this approach, the wound bed is not debrided or otherwise altered prior to repair. Despite the beveled Mohs incision, the edges of nonmarginal defects are not ''squared off'' or trimmed.

The general principles and specific operative techniques applicable to this oculofacial sector are best described with representative cases (Figs. 3.5–3.30).

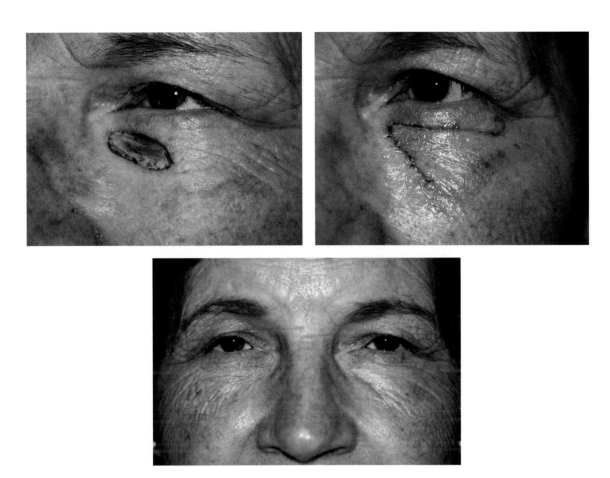

Figure 3.5

In the simplest cases, an RSTL incision is followed by flap dissection and horizontal advancement. Three weeks after surgery, incisions are blending into natural creases. (Reproduced with permission from Lippincott Williams & Wilkins. Source: Harris GJ, Perez N. Anchored flaps in post-Mohs reconstruction of the lower eyelid, cheek, and lateral canthus: avoiding eyelid distortion. Ophthal Plast Reconstr Surg 2003;19:5–13.)

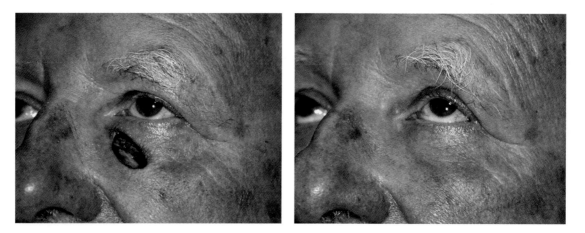

Figure 3.6

A similar case with long-term results. Closure is performed with subdermal 6-0 or 7-0 polyglactin 910 suture (knots buried) and cutaneous 7-0 nylon suture.

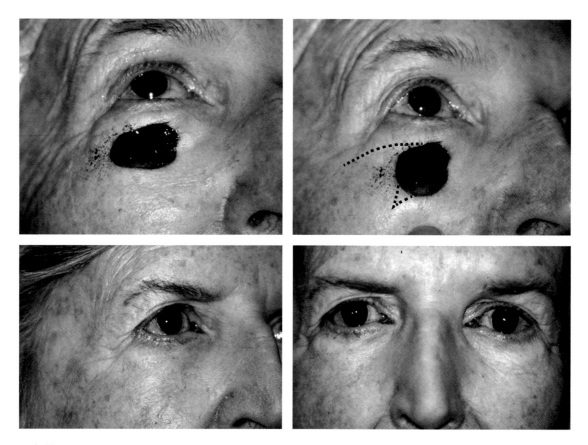

Figure 3.7

Nonmarginal Mohs defects are roughly circular, and horizontal closure creates inferior redundancy. The Burow triangle, however, can also be directed into RSTL.

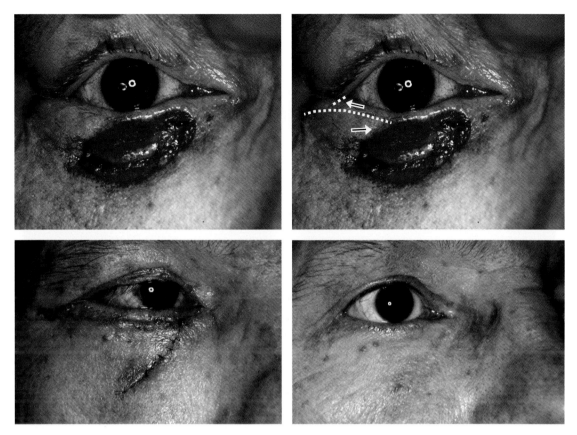

Figure 3.8

If there is even mild canthal tendon laxity, and particularly if the defect approaches the eyelid margin, horizontal tightening (upper arrow) adds stability and helps prevent ectropion. A lateral tarsal strip procedure[3] is preferred in such cases (see Figs. 3.9–3.11).

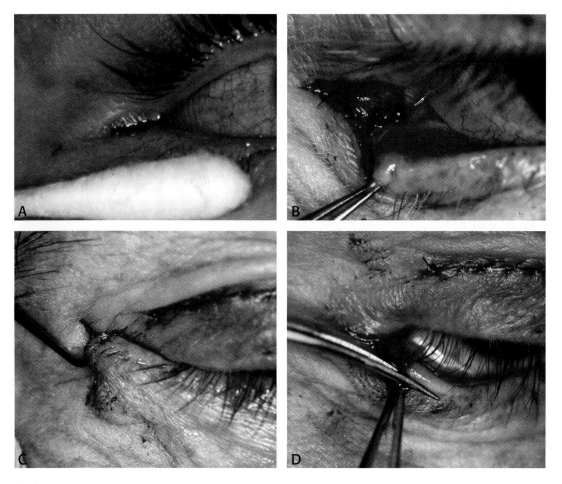

Figure 3.9

Lateral tarsal strip procedure. **A.** Horizontal incision through the skin of the lateral canthus.
B. An oblique incision through the lower limb of the lateral canthal tendon (cantholysis)
has released the eyelid. **C.** A single skin hook hangs freely from the edge of the lower eyelid;
the margin is marked where the eyelid overlaps the canthus. **D.** The mucocutaneous
junction is incised to that point.

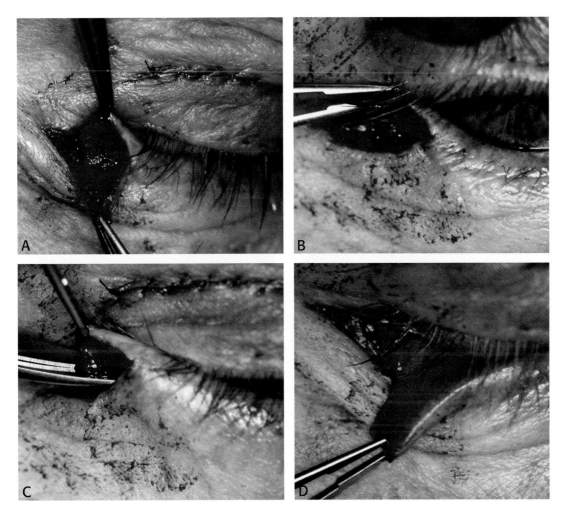

Figure 3.10

Lateral tarsal strip procedure (continued). **A.** The anterior and posterior lamellas are separated. **B.** The anterior lamella has been trimmed. When the tarsal strip procedure is used in lower eyelid reconstruction, trimming is generally limited to the ciliary margin. **C, D.** A back-cut is made in the tarsus 2.5 to 3.0 mm from the eyelid margin, creating the tarsal strip.

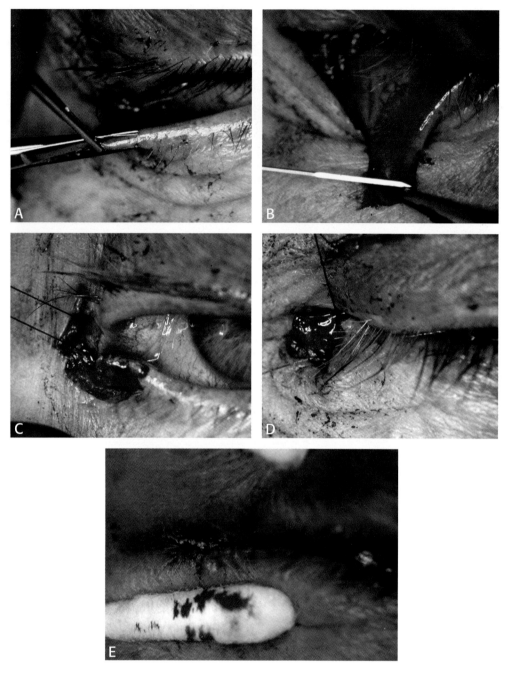

Figure 3.11

Lateral tarsal strip procedure (continued). **A.** The mucocutaneous edge of the eyelid margin is excised. **B.** The tarsal aspect is deepithelialized by scraping with a scalpel blade.
C. A double-armed 5-0 polypropylene suture (SM-1 needle) has been passed through periosteum over the orbital tubercle (on the internal aspect of the lateral orbital rim).
D. Both arms of the suture have been passed through the tarsal strip from its posterior aspect. **E.** The excess tarsus has been trimmed, the polypropylene suture tied, and the skin wound closed.

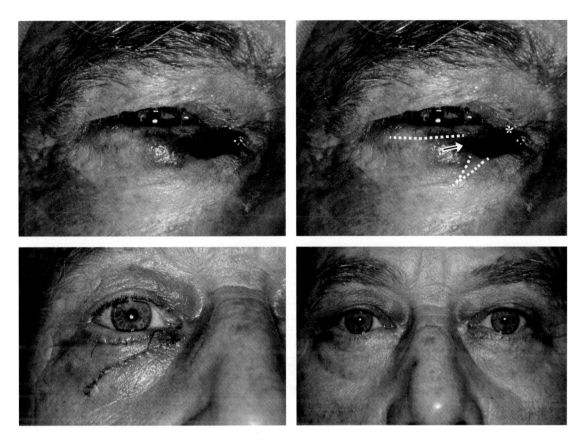

Figure 3.12

Deep anchoring protects the lower eyelid and canthal angles from flap traction. Medially, the anchor point can be the canthal tendon (asterisk), or fixed tissue inferior to it. (Modified and reproduced with permission from Lippincott Williams & Wilkins. Source: Harris GJ, Perez N. Anchored flaps in post-Mohs reconstruction of the lower eyelid, cheek, and lateral canthus: avoiding eyelid distortion. Ophthal Plast Reconstr Surg 2003; 19:5–13.)

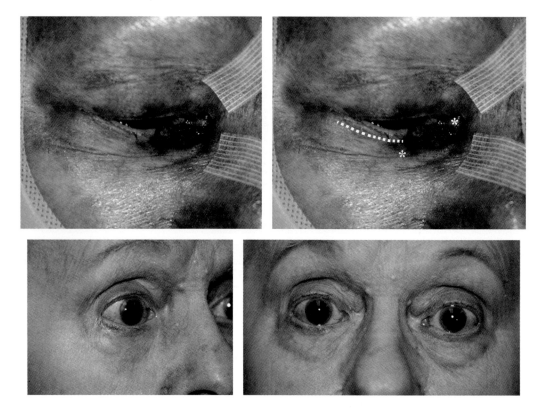

Figure 3.13

Polyglactin 910 suture, 6-0, is buried between the anterior limb of the medial canthal tendon (white asterisk) and the undersurface of the flap (yellow asterisk).

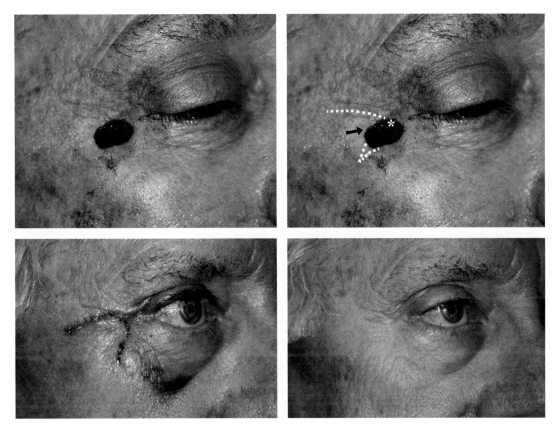

Figure 3.14

Laterally, the anchor point is periosteum over the lateral orbital rim. Simple, direct horizontal or vertical closure of even this small defect would distract the mobile canthus. Instead, a buried 5-0 polyglactin 910 suture was used to advance and anchor the subcutaneous tissue of the flap to periosteum (asterisk).

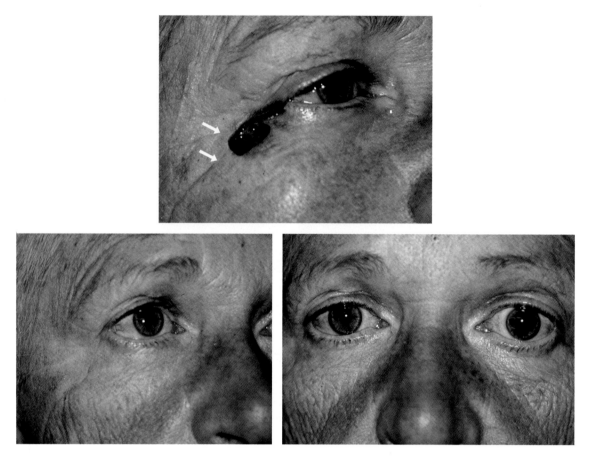

Figure 3.15

Anchored advancement flap for a lateral canthal/cheek defect. The incisions for flap dissection and dog-ear excision can often be hidden within natural creases.

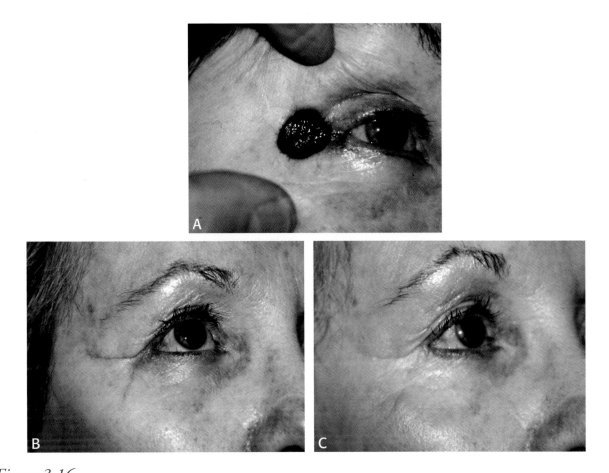

Figure 3.16

A. Lateral canthal defect for repair with an anchored advancement flap. As in other body sites, scars are most prominent 4 to 6 weeks after surgery. Patients are seen at that time, are advised to begin vitamin E oil massage, and are reassured of the long-term goals. **B.** Patient 5 weeks after surgery. **C.** Patient 6 months after surgery.

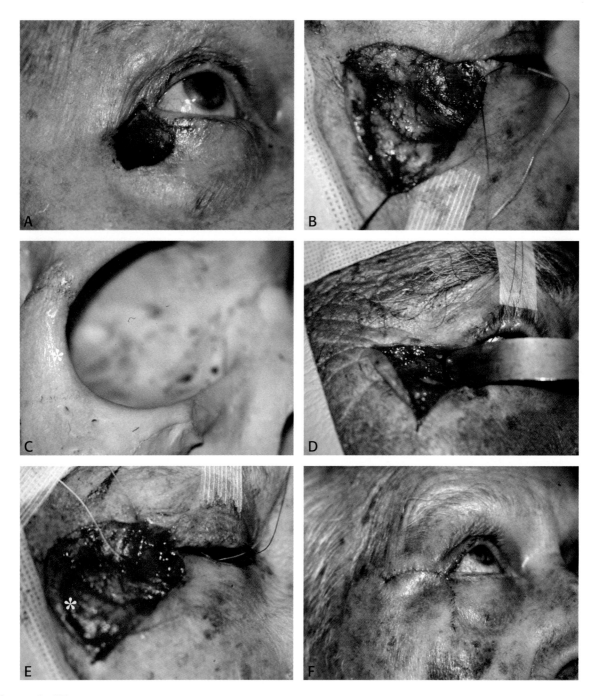

Figure 3.17

Surgical details of an anchored advancement flap. **A, B.** Dissection within subcutaneous fat avoids excessive thickness. **C, D.** Periosteum is engaged outside the lateral orbital rim (white asterisk). A retractor is held against the rim to protect the orbital septum and to prevent eyelid retraction (from the case shown in Fig. 2.14). **E, F.** An adjunctive lateral tarsal strip procedure has been performed. The flap is engaged with the anchor suture (4-0 polyglactin 910) as far laterally as necessary (yellow asterisk) to allow closure without eyelid distortion. The suture is passed in subcutaneous tissue rather than in dermis. A mild dimple may persist until the suture has been absorbed.

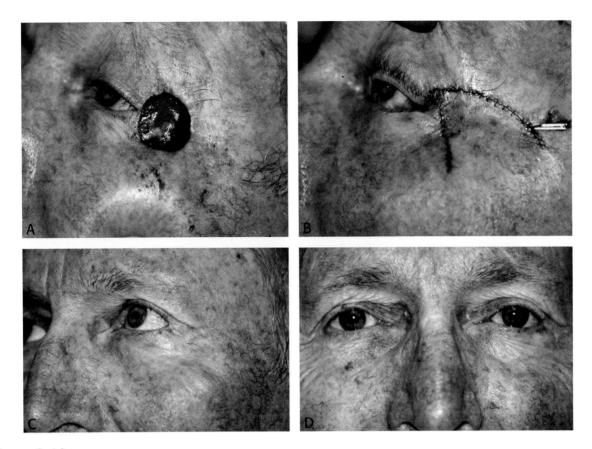

Figure 3.18

A, B. A small drain (a trimmed segment of a fluted silicone drain) is routinely placed beneath the anchored flap and sutured to the wound edge, and the eye is patched. The patient returns the morning after surgery for removal of the patch and drain. **C, D.** Patient at late follow-up. (Modified and reproduced with permission from Lippincott Williams & Wilkins. Source: Harris GJ, Perez N. Anchored flaps in post-Mohs reconstruction of the lower eyelid, cheek, and lateral canthus: avoiding eyelid distortion. Ophthal Plast Reconstr Surg 2003;19:5–13.)

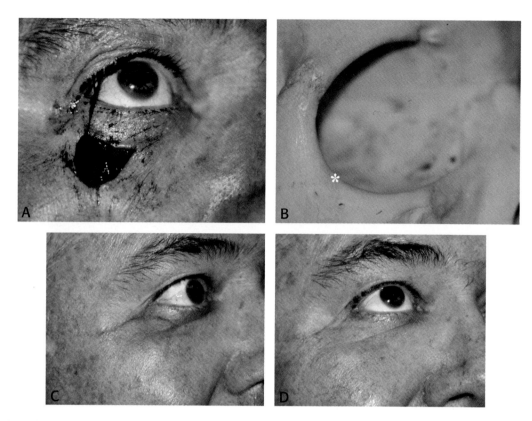

Figure 3.19

A, B. With a more inferior cheek defect, the periosteal suture is passed at the very edge of the orbital rim (asterisk) to avoid the sensory nerves that emerge from bone. **C.** Patient at 5 weeks. **D.** Patient at 5 months.

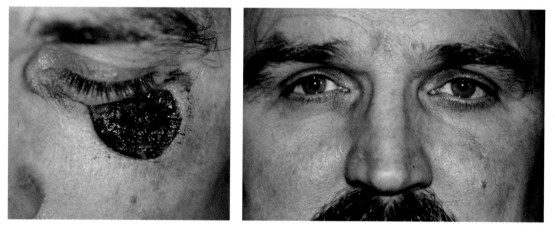

Figure 3.20

Larger cheek defect repaired with an anchored flap. Because the anchor suture stretches the skin and also protects the eyelid from that traction, the relaxing incision and flap dissection need not be as extensive as those for Mustardé cheek flaps.[4] (Reproduced with permission from Lippincott Williams & Wilkins. Source: Harris GJ, Perez N. Anchored flaps in post-Mohs reconstruction of the lower eyelid, cheek, and lateral canthus: avoiding eyelid distortion. Ophthal Plast Reconstr Surg 2003;19:5–13.)

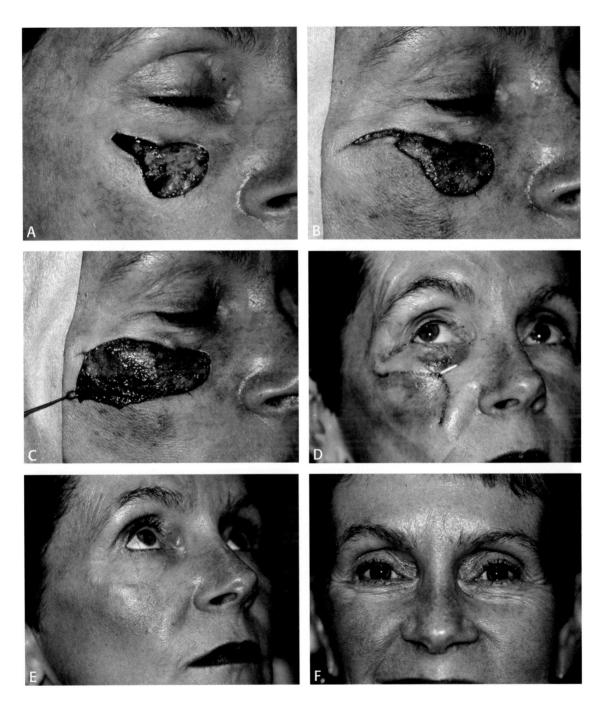

Figure 3.21

Beyond the orbital perimeter, wound beds are more fatty, skin is less elastic, and there is downward pull by deep facial muscles, all of which contribute to eyelid distortion. **A, B.** Mohs resection of a recurrent tumor included the previous scar; the relaxing incision began there. **C, D.** Deep anchoring replaces the natural osteocutaneous connections—superficial extensions of the orbitomalar and zygomatic ligaments[5,6]—that are severed in tumor removal or flap elevation. **E, F.** Patient 1 year after surgery. (Reproduced with permission from Lippincott Williams & Wilkins. Source: Harris GJ, Perez N. Anchored flaps in post-Mohs reconstruction of the lower eyelid, cheek, and lateral canthus: avoiding eyelid distortion. Ophthal Plast Reconstr Surg 2003;19:5–13.)

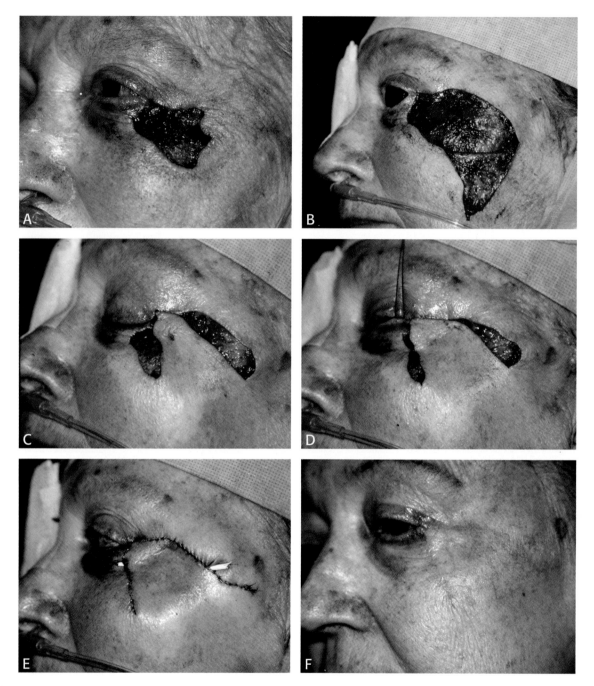

Figure 3.22

A. If a cheek defect extends to the eyelid margin or canthal angle, the risk of late distortion increases. **B–E.** In this case, eyelid skin and the cheek flap were anchored at multiple points with 4-0, 5-0, and 6-0 polyglactin 910 sutures. **F.** Early postoperative results. (Reproduced with permission from Lippincott Williams & Wilkins. Source: Harris GJ, Perez N. Anchored flaps in post-Mohs reconstruction of the lower eyelid, cheek, and lateral canthus: avoiding eyelid distortion. Ophthal Plast Reconstr Surg 2003;19:5–13.)

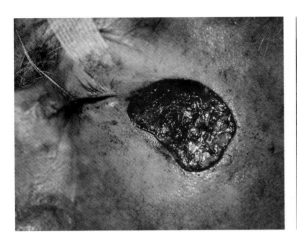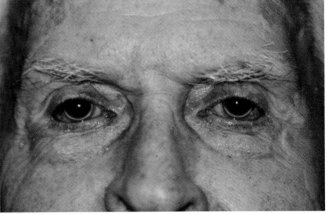

Figure 3.23

A case similar to that depicted in Figure 3.22, with longer follow-up. With broad defects, the normal, gradual transition in skin thickness is lost, and an edge may be visible.

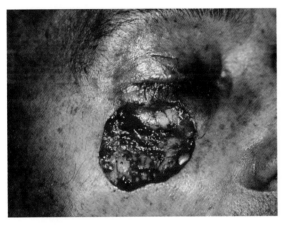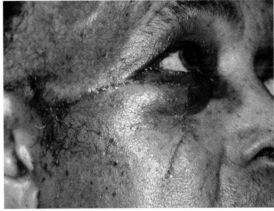

Figure 3.24

Anchored lower eyelid/cheek flap. There is no *absolute* defect size limit to this technique. If the residual skin can be stretched to close the defect completely, the tension can be mitigated with the deep anchor. (Reproduced with permission from Lippincott Williams & Wilkins. Source: Harris GJ, Perez N. Anchored flaps in post-Mohs reconstruction of the lower eyelid, cheek, and lateral canthus: avoiding eyelid distortion. Ophthal Plast Reconstr Surg 2003;19:5–13.)

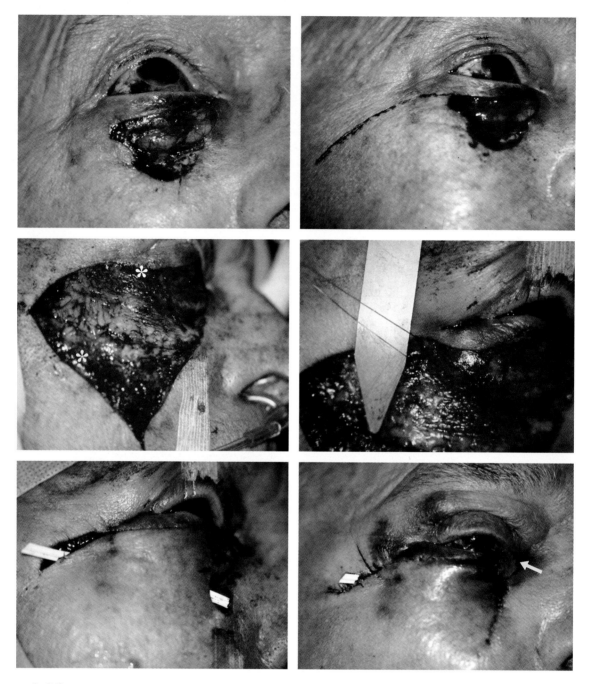

Figure 3.25

There are *relative* defect size limits to the use of a flap alone. Regardless of the extent of the relaxing incision and flap dissection, at some point intrinsic skin tension will limit advancement. This patient required a small graft (yellow arrow; see Fig. 3.26).

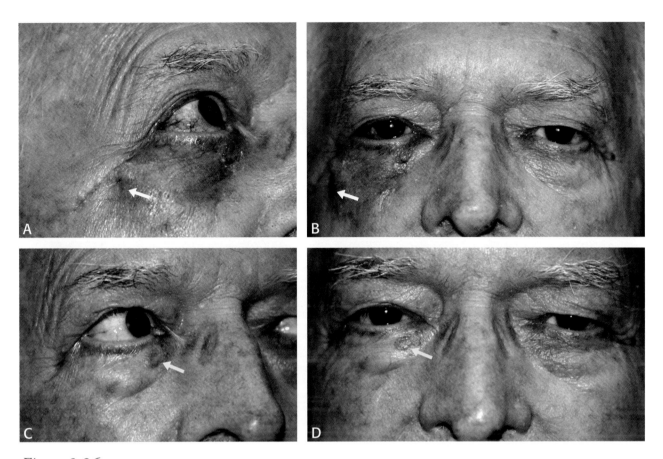

Figure 3.26

Postoperative results in the case depicted in Figure 3.25. **A, B.** Patient 3 weeks after surgery. **C, D.** Patient 7 months after surgery. With time, dimpling at the anchor site (white arrows) resolved, the flap blended well, and the graft (yellow arrows) remained obvious.

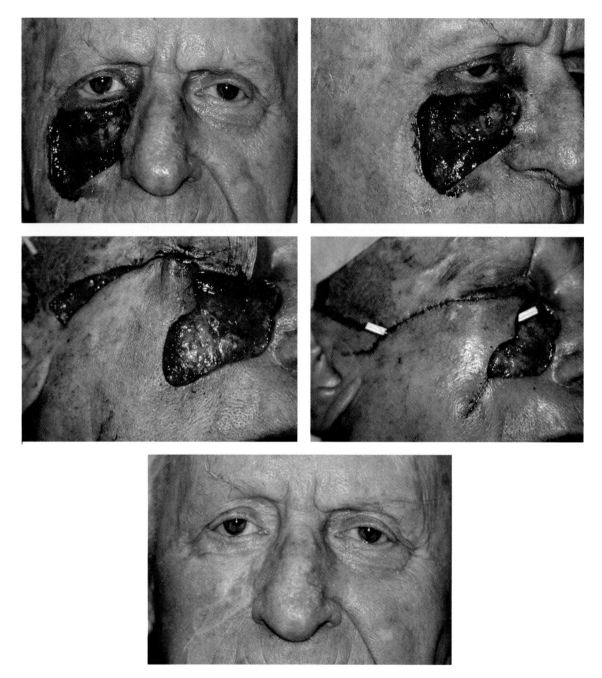

Figure 3.27

Because of the long-term drawbacks of grafting, particularly over deeper wounds, as much of the defect as possible is resurfaced with a flap. Multiple anchor points may be used. This approach reduces the size of the required skin graft—generally the more conspicuous component in late follow-up. (Modified and reproduced with permission from Lippincott Williams & Wilkins. Source: Harris GJ, Perez N. Anchored flaps in post-Mohs reconstruction of the lower eyelid, cheek, and lateral canthus: avoiding eyelid distortion. Ophthal Plast Reconstr Surg 2003;19:5–13.)

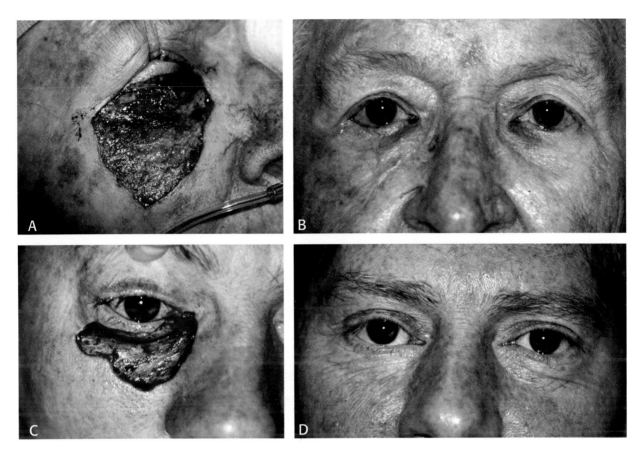

Figure 3.28

Two patients, each repaired with a wide, anchored cheek flap and a small graft (of upper eyelid skin) to the medial balance of the defect. **A, B.** An 88-year-old woman after excision of a lentigo maligna. **C, D.** A 46-year-old man after Mohs excision of a recurrent basal cell carcinoma. (Reproduced with permission from Lippincott Williams & Wilkins. Source: Harris GJ, Perez N. Anchored flaps in post-Mohs reconstruction of the lower eyelid, cheek, and lateral canthus: avoiding eyelid distortion. Ophthal Plast Reconstr Surg 2003; 19:5–13.)

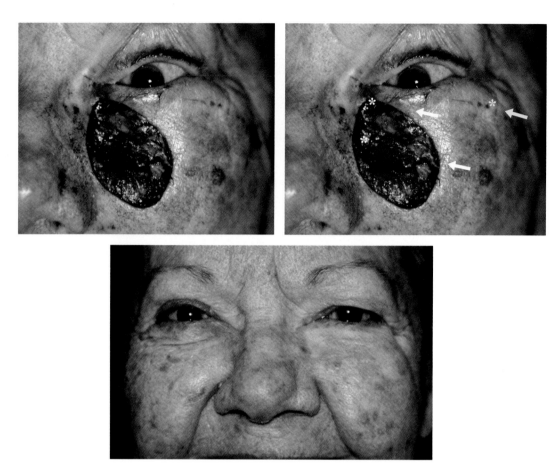

Figure 3.29

If a broad defect extends to the medial orbital rim, the flap can be anchored both medially and laterally, providing greater tissue expansion and more protection against eyelid distortion. After flap incision and elevation across the remaining eyelid and beyond the malar region, anchor sutures are placed in periosteum at the lateral rim (yellow asterisk), and in the medial canthal tendon and periosteum below it (white asterisks). The flap is placed on medial traction (with a large, double skin hook) to determine the point of lateral fixation that will permit closure without a medial graft.

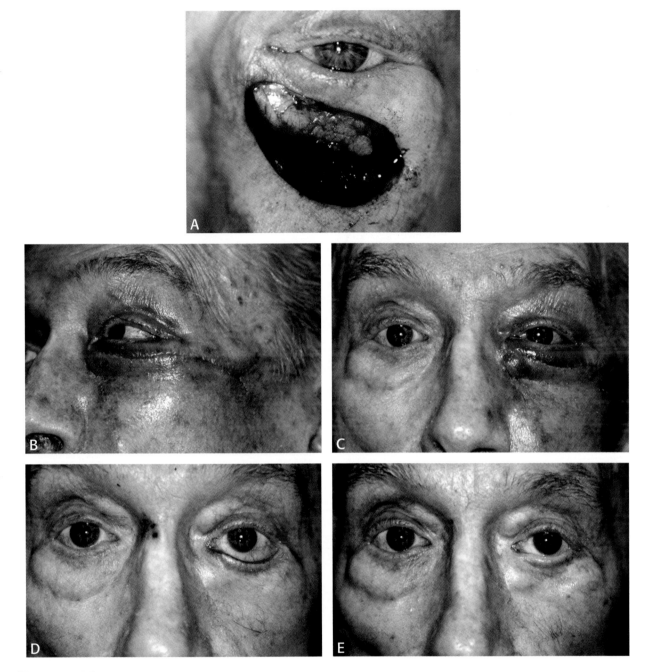

Figure 3.30

A. Extremely broad and deep defect after Mohs excision of a recurrent basal cell carcinoma.
B, C. Patient 1 week after surgery, which included a prophylactic tarsal strip procedure and
a wide cheek flap anchored both laterally and medially. **D, E.** Despite these measures,
wound bed fibrosis caused lower eyelid retraction, which was corrected secondarily with a
postauricular skin graft and a small, permanent lateral tarsorrhaphy.

References

1. Borges AF. Relaxed skin tension lines (RSTL) versus other skin lines. Plast Reconstr Surg 1984;73:144–150.
2. Harris GJ, Perez N. Anchored flaps in post-Mohs reconstruction of the lower eyelid, cheek, and lateral canthus: avoiding eyelid distortion. Ophthal Plast Reconstr Surg 2003;19:5–13.
3. Anderson RL, Gordy DD. The tarsal strip procedure. Arch Ophthalmol 1979;97:2192–2196.
4. Mustardé JC. Repair and Reconstruction in the Orbital Region. 2nd Ed. Edinburgh: Churchill Livingstone, 1980:52–57.
5. Kikkawa DO, Lemke BN, Dortzbach RK. Relations of the superficial musculoaponeurotic system to the orbit and characterization of the orbitomalar ligament. Ophthal Plast Reconstr Surg 1996;12:77–88.
6. Lucarelli MJ, Khwarg SI, Lemke BN, et al. The anatomy of midfacial ptosis. Ophthal Plast Reconstr Surg 2000;16:7–22.

Nonmarginal Defects of the Medial Canthal Region

Among the oculofacial sectors, the medial canthal region presents unique reconstructive challenges. Multiple components—differing in skin thickness, contour, and relative mobility—converge in a concavity. For practical purposes, these components might be viewed as contributions from four aesthetic units: the upper eyelid; the lower eyelid; and the nasal sidewall, both above and below the level of the medial commissure (Fig. 4.1). Not surprisingly, tumor growth does not respect these aesthetic boundaries (Fig. 4.2).

Skin grafting of the medial canthus may be an acceptable option in young, non-Mohs patients with benign, superficial lesions (Figs. 4.3). When skin cancers have been removed by Mohs surgery, however, free grafts have limitations beyond the common concerns of color and thickness mismatch. Wound bed vascularity (and graft survival) may be compromised because of prior surgery, radiation, cryosurgery, or electrodissection. If a tumor-free defect extends to bare bone, the bed will be similarly inhospitable for grafting. Relatively heavy cautery during the tumor resection in this nexus of major vessels can accentuate postoperative wound bed contraction. As a result, an appropriate-size graft at the time of reconstruction may become heaped-up or corrugated during the ensuing 6 to 8 weeks (Fig. 4.4).

Other reconstructive choices for the medial canthus have included spontaneous granulation (the *laissez-faire* technique).[1] In this concavity, however, with loose eyelid skin adjacent to fixed nasal skin, scar contraction can convert an *arc* to a *chord* within the operative site and draw in loose eyelid skin from beyond the site (Fig. 4.5). Single large flaps that cross aesthetic unit boundaries can cause similar webbing. Flaps derived from the midline or paramedian forehead bring in thick tissue clearly distinct from the neighboring eyelid skin.

With a postoperative goal of preserving the canthal concavity, my preference is to combine local flaps derived from the residual skin of each involved medial canthal component or aesthetic unit, and to use the anterior limb of the canthal tendon or more inferior fixed tissue as the underpinning for the reconstruction[2] (Figs. 4.6 and 4.7).

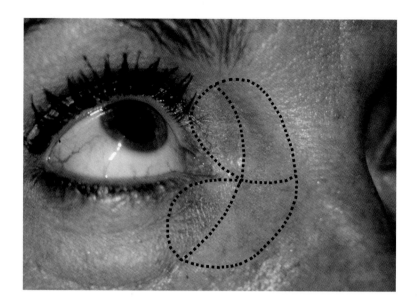

Figure 4.1

The medial canthal region represents the convergence of multiple aesthetic units that differ in contour, skin thickness, and relative mobility.

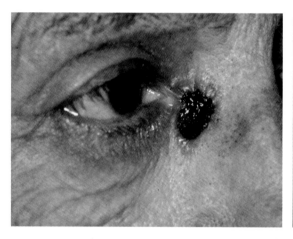
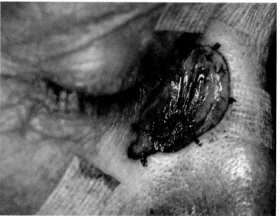

Figure 4.2

Medial canthal basal cell carcinoma before and after Mohs excision. Tumor growth extends across aesthetic units.

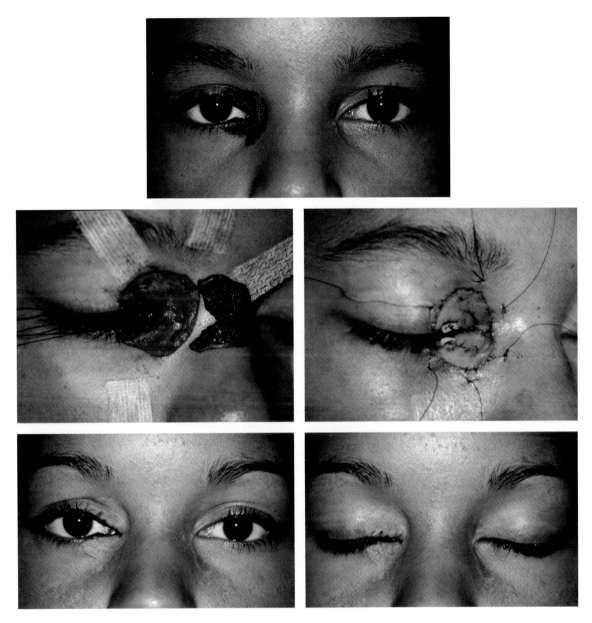

Figure 4.3

Benign nevus in a young girl, excised and resurfaced with a postauricular skin graft. One-year postoperative appearance, with some thickness disparity.

Figure 4.4

Skin graft corrugation and irregularity followed late wound bed fibrosis and contraction.

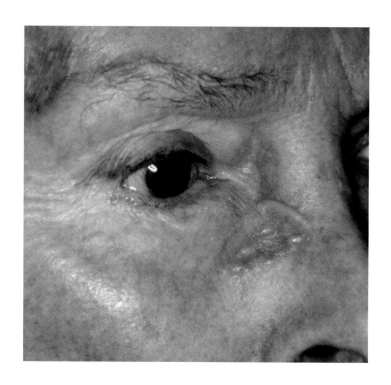

Figure 4.5

Medial canthal webbing followed nondirected healing after tumor excision.

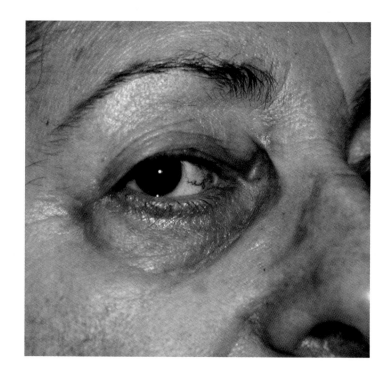

Figure 4.6

When planning medial canthal reconstruction, defects are first viewed in terms of their aesthetic unit components. After flaps are developed from the edge of each involved unit, they are anchored individually to the canthal tendon or to more inferior deep connective tissue.

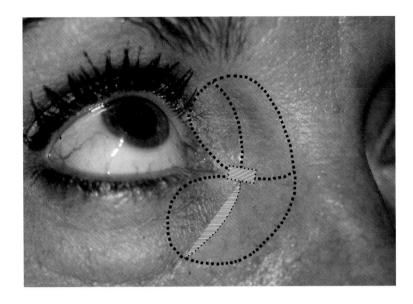

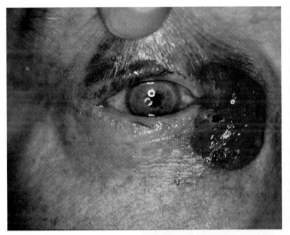

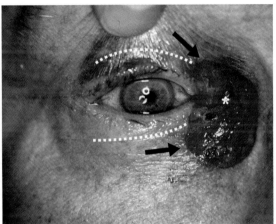

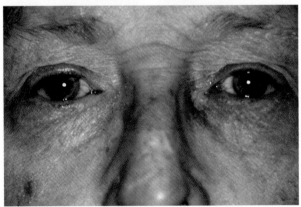

Figure 4.7

Flaps derived from the periphery of each component of the defect—here, the upper and lower eyelids—are fixed independently to the tendon (asterisk) with subcutaneous sutures. Postoperatively, the canthal concavity is preserved. (Reproduced with permission from Lippincott Williams & Wilkins. Source: Harris GJ, Logani, SC. Multiple aesthetic unit flaps for medial canthal reconstruction. Ophthal Plast Reconstr Surg 1998;14:352–359.)

Medial canthal defects vary in size and relative involvement of each aesthetic unit. As in other sectors, the reconstructive options for a defect of any given size differ with the distensibility of the patient's residual tissucs. For these reasons, no single formula is applicable to every case. Some general guidelines are applied as defect size increases: a shift from simple advancement sutures to advancement flaps; the addition of more flaps per case; particular caution at the upper eyelid/glabellar junction if there is intact canthal skin inferior to the defect; the introduction of grafts, sparingly and begrudgingly, as necessary final elements; and a combination of techniques used in the medial canthal sector and the lower eyelid/cheek/lateral canthal sector (see Chapter 3) for large defects that bridge the two. These general principles and specific operative procedures are best described with representative cases of increasing complexity (Figs. 4.8–4.28).

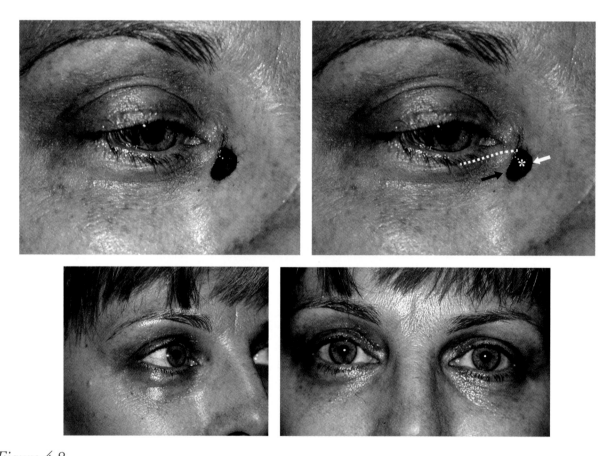

Figure 4.8

Small defect bridging aesthetic units. Simple, direct approximation might cause a web. Instead, a small lower eyelid flap and the nasal sidewall edge (without a relaxing incision) are each anchored to periosteum (asterisk) with subdermal polyglactin 910 suture. Skin is closed with 7-0 nylon suture.

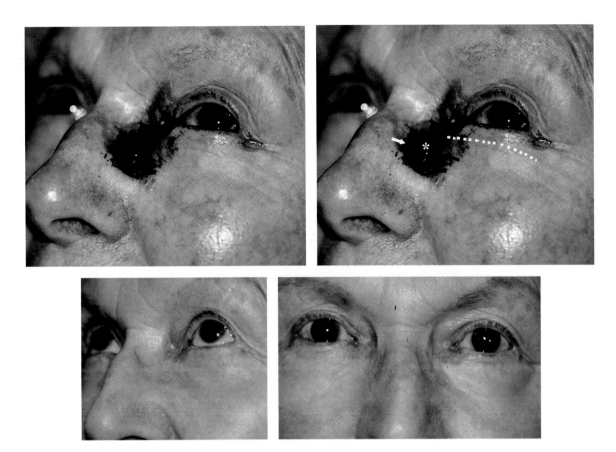

Figure 4.9

Larger defect in similar location. Distensibility of the nasal skin allowed similar repair (subdermal 5-0 polyglactin 910 suture on the nasal edge and 6-0 on the eyelid flap, each anchored to deep tissue). Redundancies above and below are excised as necessary.

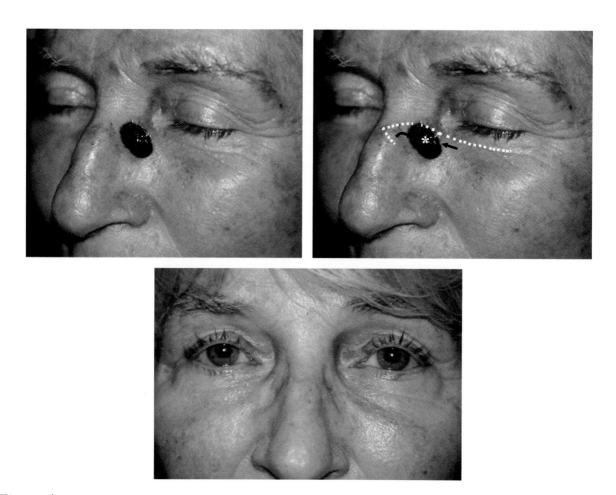

Figure 4.10

With less distensible skin, or a larger defect, a nasal *flap* is added—here, a V-to-Y rotation flap—and both flaps are anchored deeply.

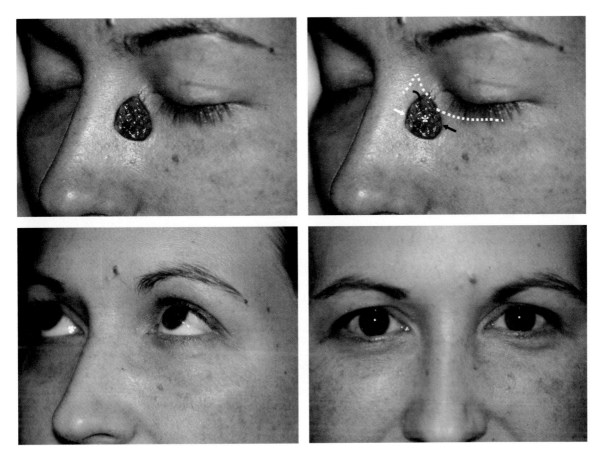

Figure 4.11

A young patient treated with medial edge advancement, a small rotation flap from above, and an advancement flap from the lower eyelid—all anchored to periosteum.

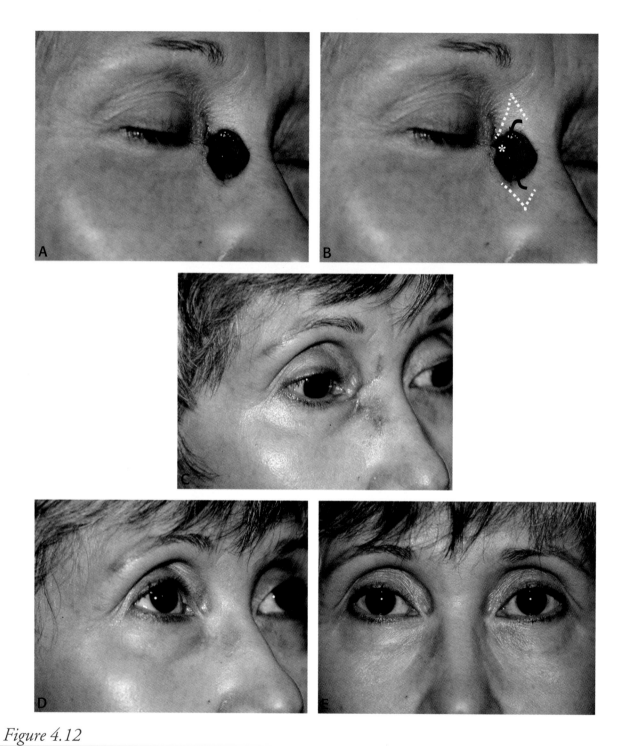

Figure 4.12

A, B. For a defect above and below the level of tendon, corresponding nasal sidewall flaps are apposed and anchored. **C.** Patient 1 week after surgery. **D, E.** Patient several months later.

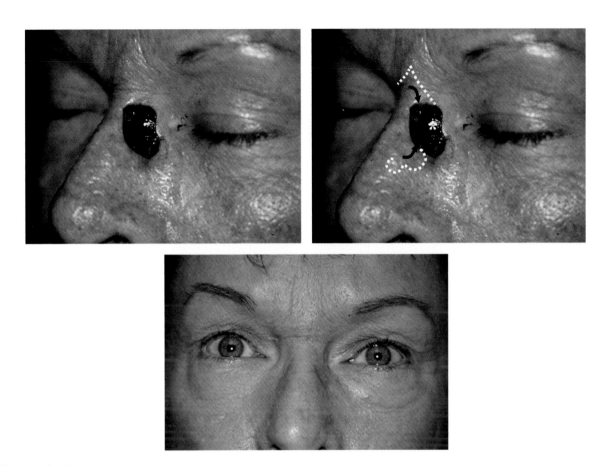

Figure 4.13

A bilobed flap was used inferiorly, but flap shape may be less important than respecting aesthetic unit boundaries and anchoring to fixed tissue.

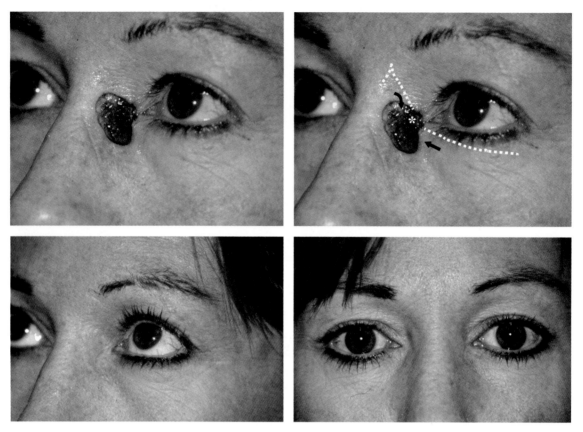

Figure 4.14

The fundamental principle for a medium-size, superficial defect—here, the combination of glabellar and lower eyelid flaps—can be extended to larger, deeper defects (see Fig. 4.15).

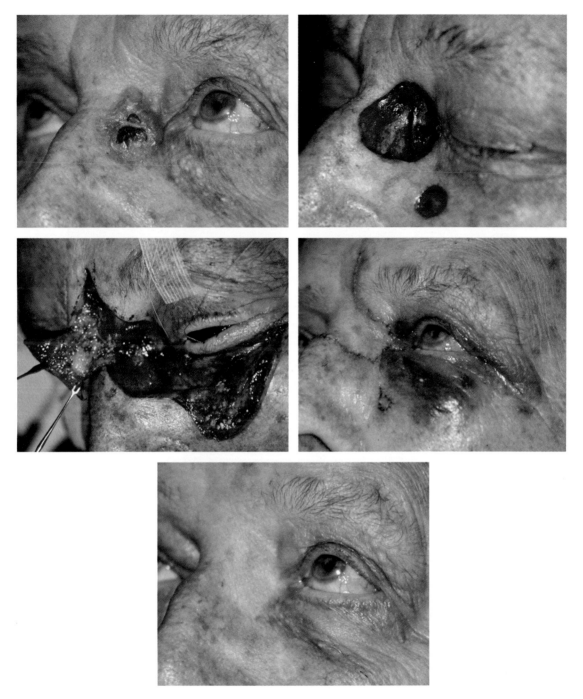

Figure 4.15

Had this deep defect been resurfaced with a graft thin enough to survive, a depression would have resulted. Instead, anchored glabellar and lower eyelid flaps produced a satisfactory thickness match. (Color discontinuity reflects the patient's preoperative pigmentary mottling.)

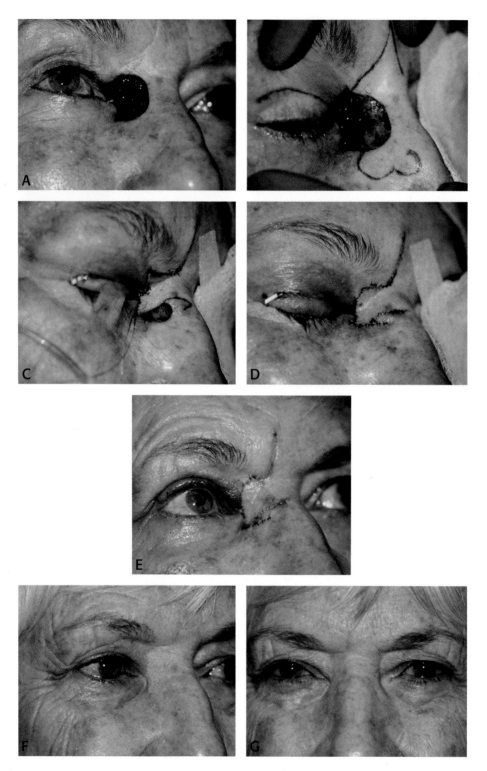

Figure 4.16

A–D. A tentative plan—here, for three large flaps—is useful, but committing to all flaps with simultaneous incisions is not advised. Transposition of the first one or two flaps may achieve more than anticipated, allowing the plan to be modified. The patient 1 week **(E)** and 6 months **(F, G)** after surgery.

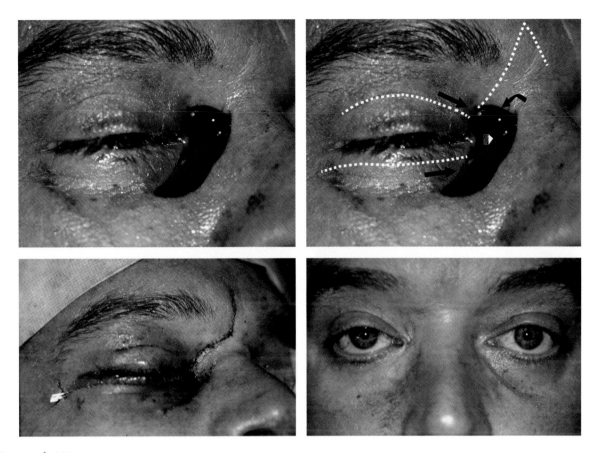

Figure 4.17

Mohs resection of a basal cell carcinoma that had recurred under a skin graft included removal of the medial canthal tendon and part of the lacrimal sac. Reconstruction included lacrimal intubation and placement of a Mitek microanchor (Mitek Surgical Products, Westwood, MA) as the fixation point for each of the three flaps.

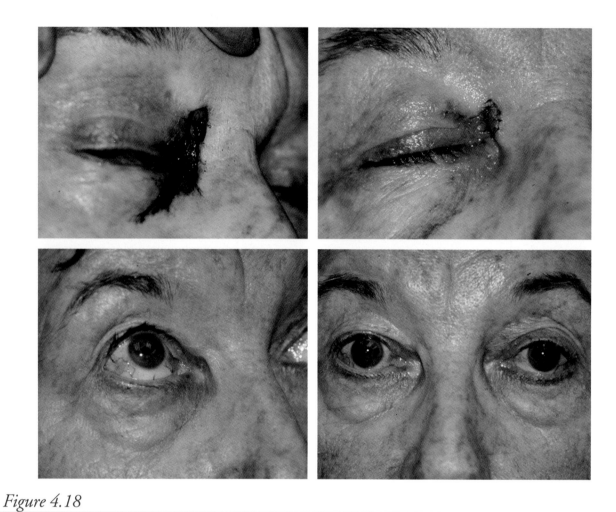

Figure 4.18

A medial canthal "danger zone," in which even small defects are at high risk for webbing, is the junction of loose upper eyelid skin and fixed glabellar skin. In addition, an upper eyelid web may continue inferiorly as an epicanthal fold if the skin below the defect is lax. Here, a single rhomboid flap crossed the eyelid–glabellar junction, violating the aesthetic unit principle (see Figs. 4.19–4.21).

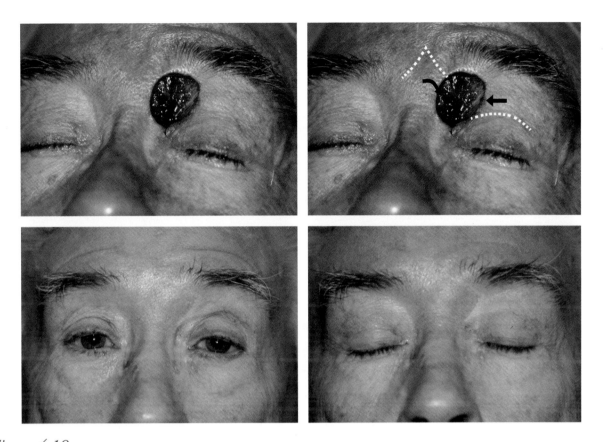

Figure 4.19

Combined glabellar and upper eyelid flaps can reduce, but not eliminate, the risk of webbing in this region. Anchoring the glabellar flap avoids transmission of that flap's tension, but it may be difficult to identify an anchor point in more superior defects. Wound bed fibrosis in the eyelid component remains a source of traction on lax eyelid skin lateral to the defect.

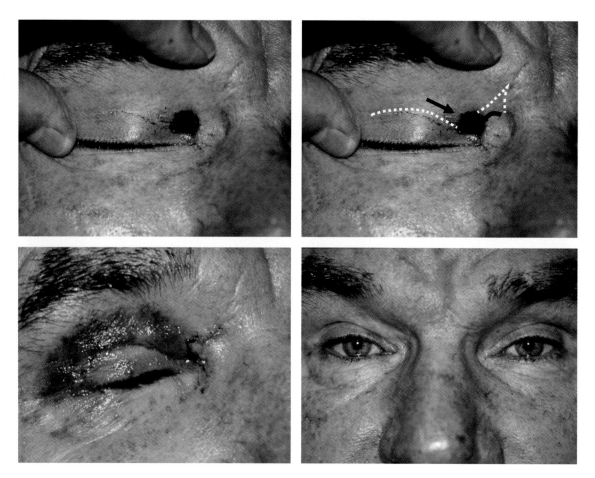

Figure 4.20

Combined glabellar and upper eyelid flaps in the "danger zone." A long eyelid crease incision, wide dissection, and medial advancement of the flap with each suture bite will recruit more skin into the defect, while reducing the lateral laxity that contributes to the deformity.

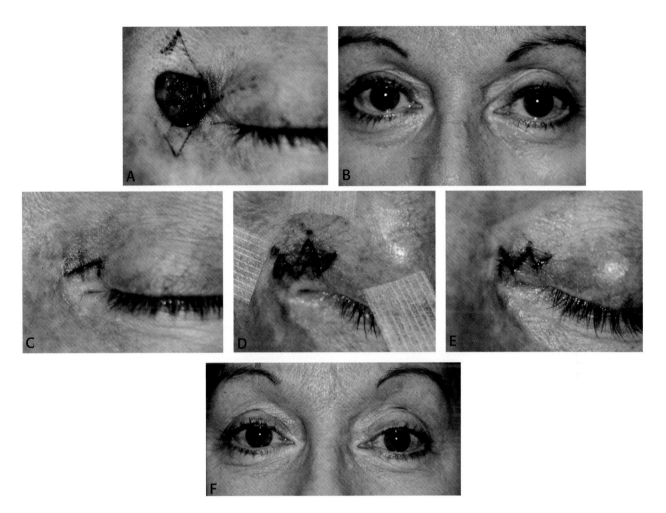

Figure 4.21

If late webbing does occur, Z-plasty wound revision is possible. **A.** A defect involving the glabellar aspect of the left nasal sidewall and a portion of the upper eyelid was repaired with anchored, opposing V-to-Y flaps and an upper eyelid flap. **B.** One year after reconstruction, a band is visible. (A small free graft over the eyelid component would have been an alternative to the eyelid flap, but passive contraction of the graft over the wound bed might have produced a similar outcome.) **C–E.** Double Z-plasty revision lengthens the contracted band by redistributing tension across the concavity. **F.** Patient 4 months after revision of the canthal band.

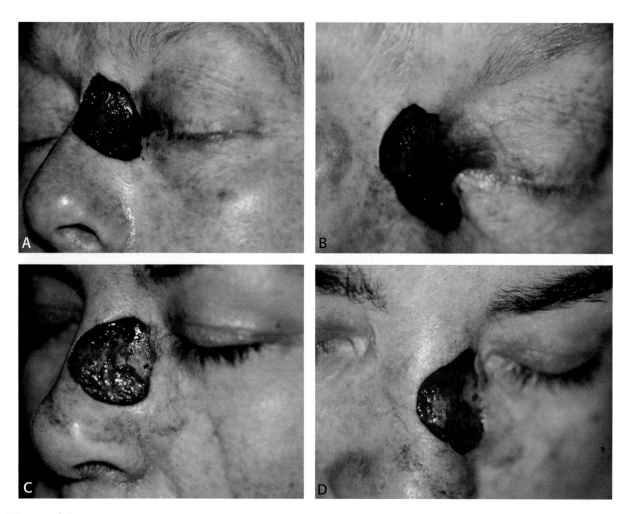

Figure 4.22

Two women **(A, B; C, D)** with large defects primarily involving the nasal sidewall component of the medial canthal region. If staged axial forehead flaps were elected, the rotated tips would be excessively thick; large, thin skin grafts would leave prominent depressions (see Figs. 4.23 and 4.24).

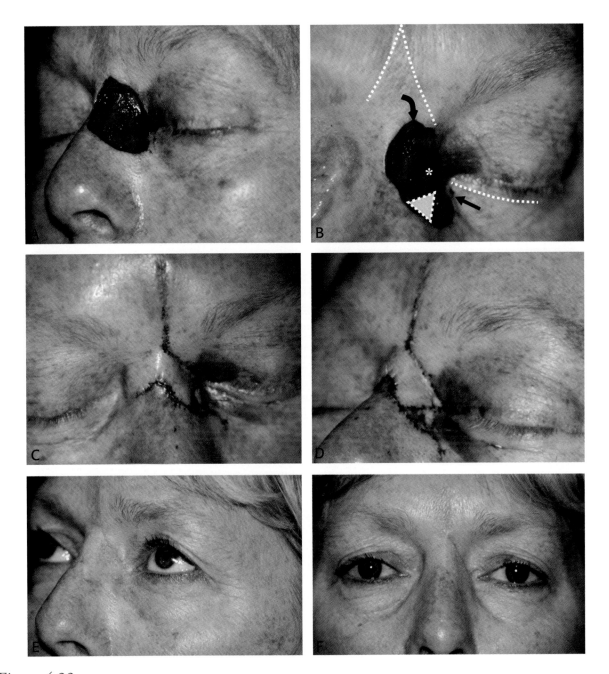

Figure 4.23

A–D. In this patient the defect was downsized with local anchored flaps, and the small balance was resurfaced with a graft (redundancy of the advanced flaps). **E, F.** The patient 5 months after surgery. (Fair-skinned patients are reassured that incisional scars will continue to fade for up to a year, and that the absence of distortion in the short term is generally permanent.)

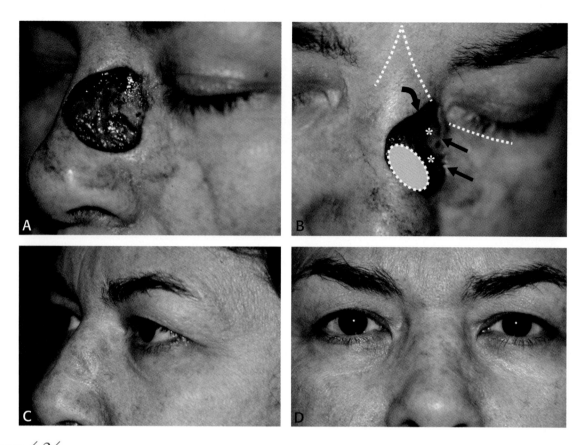

Figure 4.24

A, B. In this similar case, the defect was downsized with local flaps anchored at multiple points, and the balance was grafted with postauricular skin. **C, D.** The patient 1 year after surgery, with a small depression in the area of the thinner graft.

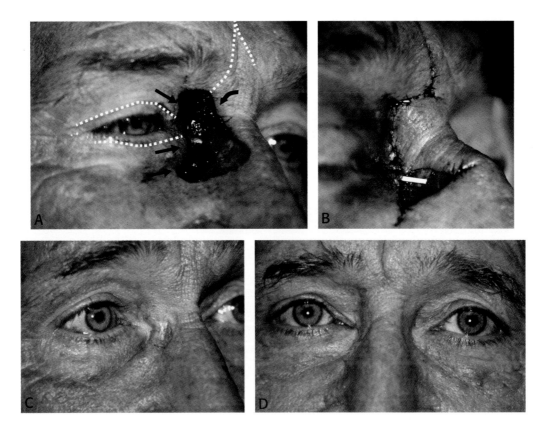

Figure 4.25

A. A defect after Mohs excision of a basal cell carcinoma that had recurred after primary radiotherapy. Three large flaps were advanced and anchored to the canthal tendon (exposed in the wound bed). **B.** Grafting is the final step after the defect has been downsized maximally. (The lower eyelid flap drain is visible in the graft bed.) **C, D.** Patient at late follow-up. (Reproduced with permission from Lippincott Williams & Wilkins. Source: Harris GJ, Logani, SC. Multiple aesthetic unit flaps for medial canthal reconstruction. Ophthal Plast Reconstr Surg 1998;14:352–359.)

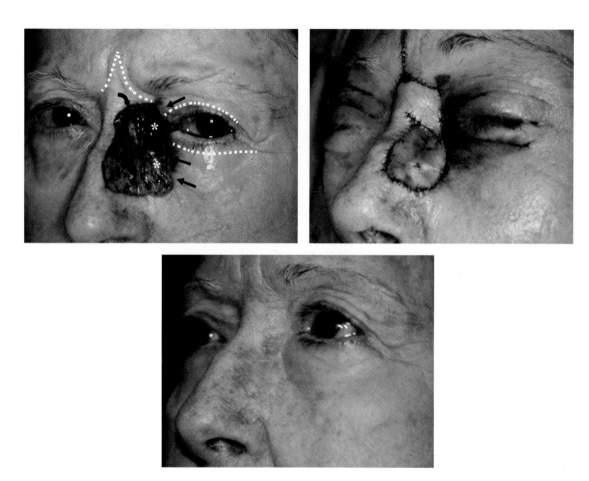

Figure 4.26

Defect after Mohs resection of a basal cell carcinoma that recurred after multiple prior surgeries. Whenever possible, grafts are restricted to the more rigid nasal sidewall, where there is less shrinkage during wound bed fibrosis. (Reproduced with permission from Lippincott Williams & Wilkins. Source: Harris GJ, Logani, SC. Multiple aesthetic unit flaps for medial canthal reconstruction. Ophthal Plast Reconstr Surg 1998;14:352–359.)

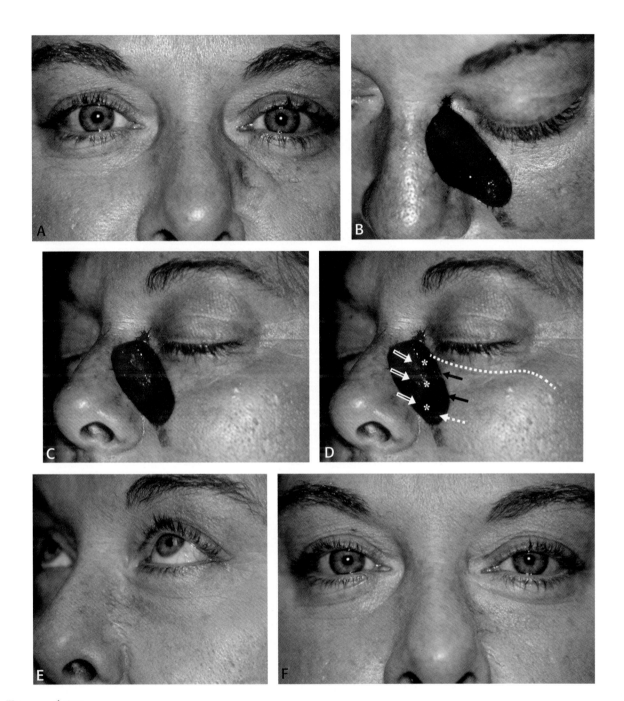

Figure 4.27

A. A young woman with thick, inelastic skin and a deeply invasive basal cell carcinoma.
B, C. Post-Mohs defect of the nasal sidewall, lower eyelid, and cheek. **D.** The nasal edge
was advanced with multiple subcutaneous-to-periosteal polyglactin 910 sutures. The lower
eyelid/cheek skin and subcutaneous tissue were elevated as a flap, cheek fat was advanced to
shallow the defect, and the eyelid/cheek flap was advanced and anchored to approximate
the nasal edge. **E, F.** Although not perfect, the late result is preferable to that expected with
a thick forehead flap or a thin graft.

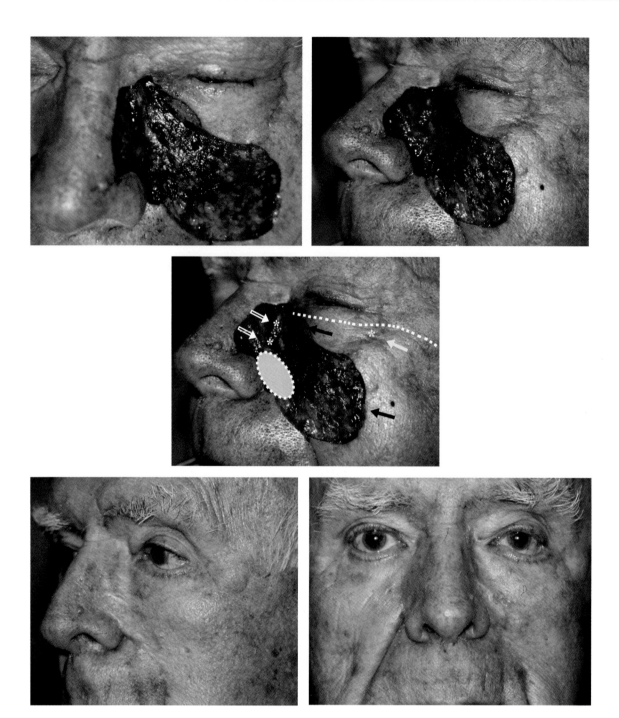

Figure 4.28

For large defects that bridge the medial canthal and the lower eyelid/cheek sectors, the techniques used in each region are combined. In this case, a single large graft was avoided because contraction over the heavily cauterized, fatty wound bed was anticipated. Instead, the defect was narrowed with a cheek flap anchored at both the lateral and medial orbital rims, the nasal sidewall was advanced with deep fixation, and the balance was grafted. A prophylactic lateral tarsal strip procedure was also performed. At late follow-up, there is mild lower eyelid retraction; the grafted portion remains most visible.

References

1. Harrington JH. Reconstruction of the medial canthus by spontaneous granulation (laissez-faire): a review. Ann Ophthalmol 1982;14:956–970.
2. Harris GJ, Logani SC. Multiple aesthetic unit flaps for medial canthal reconstruction. Ophthal Plast Reconstr Surg 1998;14:352–359.

Nonmarginal Defects of the Upper Eyelid, Eyebrow, Glabella, Forehead, and Temple

*T*he uppermost oculofacial sector includes the eyebrows, interbrow glabellar region, forehead, and temples (Fig. 1.4). In contrast to the multiple aesthetic units of the medial canthal region, these components share similarities of dermal thickness and subcutaneous fat, and underlying muscle action produces mass movements of the entire sector. Although the region can be considered a single aesthetic unit, variations in defect size and position within the unit may raise different concerns. These include the continuity of each eyebrow, positional symmetry of the eyebrow pair, maintenance of the normal hairline, symmetry of the upper eyelid folds and supratarsal sulci, and camouflage of incisional scars in a highly visible area.

In this sector, reconstruction with skin grafts has the same limitations of color and thickness mismatch, late contraction, and corrugation discussed in earlier chapters. The results with large rotational flaps also may be less than ideal (Fig. 5.1).

In this region, the reconstructive options might be arranged in a scale, which provides progressively more tissue, but at an increasing aesthetic cost (Fig. 5.2). The latter judgment considers the transverse direction of RSTL in the sector, skin color and thickness, and the multiple stages and months-long distortion of tissue expansion. With these considerations, our reconstructive goal in this sector is to exploit direct approximation and advancement flaps fully before resorting to less aesthetic alternatives[1] (Fig. 5.3).

Thus far, ascension of the reconstructive scale to tissue expansion or microvascular transfer has not been needed in the repair of post-Mohs defects. Although these techniques would be difficult to use in primary

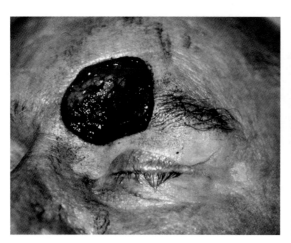
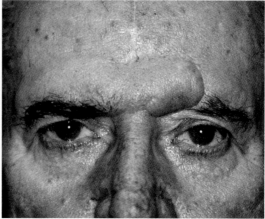

Figure 5.1

Glabellar/forehead/eyebrow defect repaired with a midline forehead flap. The long curvilinear scars and thick skin are prone to pincushion deformity that may need revision. (Reproduced with permission from Lippincott Williams & Wilkins. Source: Harris GJ, Garcia GH. Advancement flaps for large defects of the eyebrow, glabella, forehead and temple. Ophthal Plast Reconstr Surg 2002;18:138–145.)

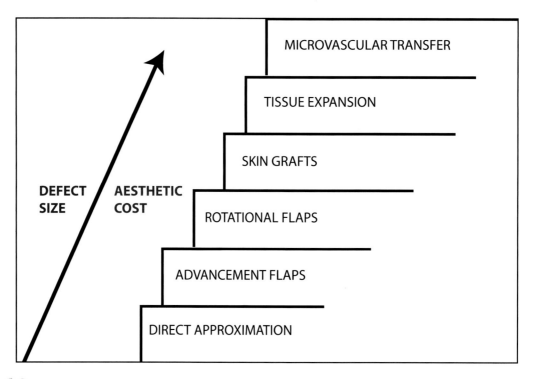

Figure 5.2

Reconstructive options for defects of the glabella, eyebrow, forehead, and temple. Ascending the scale provides progressively more tissue, but at a higher aesthetic cost. (Modified with permission from Lippincott Williams & Wilkins. Source: Harris GJ, Garcia GH. Advancement flaps for large defects of the eyebrow, glabella, forehead and temple. Ophthal Plast Reconstr Surg 2002;18:138–145.)

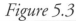

Figure 5.3

Preferred thresholds for reconstructive options, maximizing direct approximation and advancement flaps before moving up the scale. (Modified with permission from Lippincott Williams & Wilkins. Source: Harris GJ, Garcia GH. Advancement flaps for large defects of the eyebrow, glabella, forehead and temple. Ophthal Plast Reconstr Surg 2002;18:138–145.)

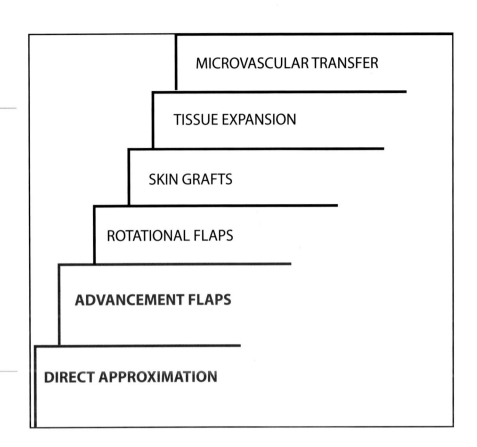

reconstruction, extremely large defects in this oculofacial sector could be resurfaced temporarily with split-thickness skin grafts, and later revised. Tissue expansion over the broad frontal bone is highly effective, but involves a several-month period of distortion.

For completeness, the nonmarginal upper eyelids are included in this oculofacial sector. As noted in Chapter 2, basal cell carcinomas of the upper eyelid margin are far less common than those of the lower eyelid margin. Isolated *non*marginal upper eyelid tumors may be even less common. In my experience, this area is more likely to be involved in continuity with the eyebrow, glabella, or temple. Reconstructive goals for the eyelid portion of defects that span these sites include thinner skin and greater mobility.

The general approach and specific techniques used in this sector are depicted in the following representative cases (Figs. 5.4–5.21).

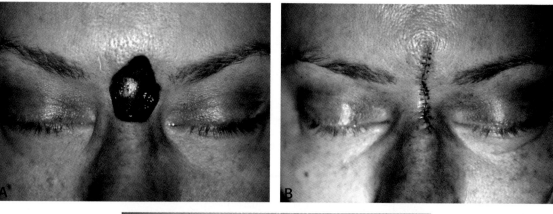

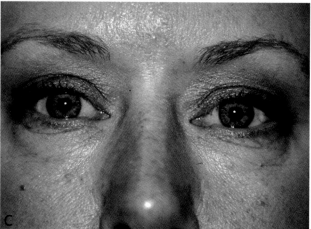

Figure 5.4

A. A large, midline glabellar defect after Mohs resection of an eccrine carcinoma. **B.** Repair included substantial subdermal approximation (without undermining) and plucking of medial brow hairs. **C.** Patient 7 months after surgery. (Reproduced with permission from Lippincott Williams & Wilkins. Source: Harris GJ, Garcia GH. Advancement flaps for large defects of the eyebrow, glabella, forehead and temple. Ophthal Plast Reconstr Surg 2002;18:138–145.)

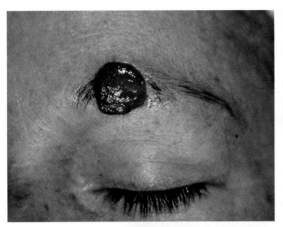 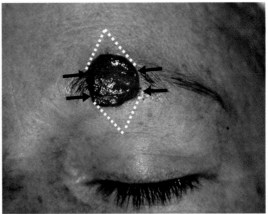

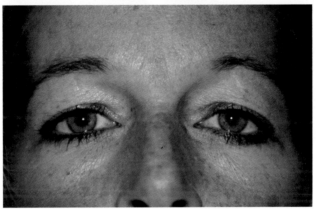

Figure 5.5

Small eyebrow defect. Standard techniques include alignment of the highest and lowest rows of brow hairs and excision of Burow triangles. Although the scar is oblique to the RSTL, the primary objective—restoration of brow continuity—is satisfied, and the upper eyelid fold is unaltered. (Modified and reproduced with permission from Lippincott Williams & Wilkins. Source: Harris GJ, Garcia GH. Advancement flaps for large defects of the eyebrow, glabella, forehead and temple. Ophthal Plast Reconstr Surg 2002;18: 138–145.)

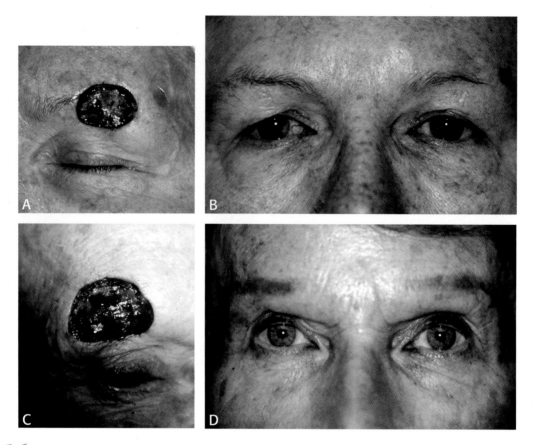

Figure 5.6

Medium **(A, B)** and large **(C, D)** eyebrow defects can be directly approximated in the manner shown in Figure 5.5, without interpolating bulky flaps or patch grafts. The hair deficit is shifted laterally, where it is more easily camouflaged with an eyebrow pencil. (Reproduced with permission from Lippincott Williams & Wilkins. Source: Harris GJ, Garcia GH. Advancement flaps for large defects of the eyebrow, glabella, forehead and temple. Ophthal Plast Reconstr Surg 2002;18:138–145.)

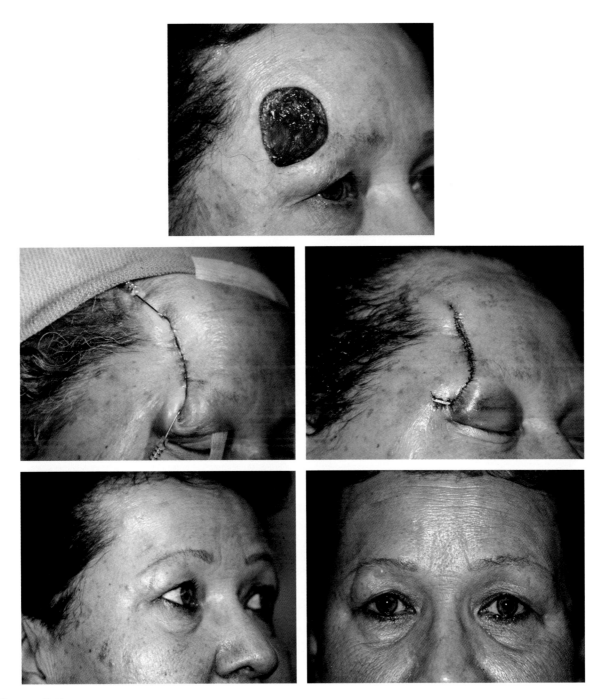

Figure 5.7

Large eyebrow/forehead defect after staged resection of a lentigo maligna melanoma. Edges were advanced directly with subdermal 4-0 and 5-0 polyglactin 910 sutures, and superior and inferior redundancies were excised. Horizontal approximation preserves eyebrow alignment at the relatively minor cost of an anti-RSTL scar. (Although not elected thus far, W-plasty revision is an option in such cases). (Reproduced with permission from Lippincott Williams & Wilkins. Source: Harris GJ, Garcia GH. Advancement flaps for large defects of the eyebrow, glabella, forehead and temple. Ophthal Plast Reconstr Surg 2002;18:138–145.)

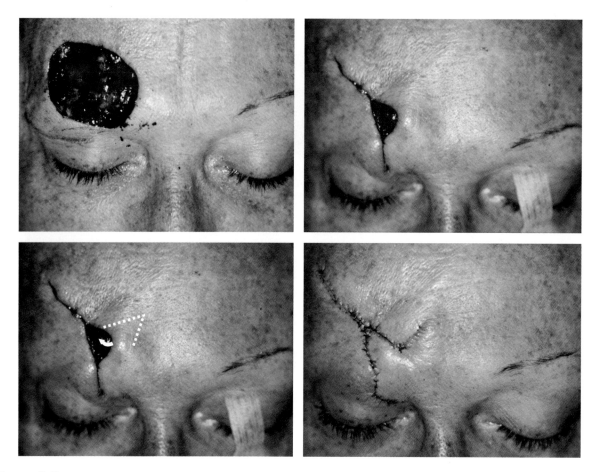

Figure 5.8

Large eyebrow/forehead defect. If defect size exceeds the relative limits of horizontal advancement, other reconstructive options can often *supplement* the technique, rather than serve as the primary methods of repair. In this case, a large rotational flap could have resurfaced the entire defect. Instead, the wound edges were advanced maximally, generating vertical excess that was rotated to fill the deficit (see Fig. 5.9). (Modified and reproduced with permission from Lippincott Williams & Wilkins. Source: Harris GJ, Garcia GH. Advancement flaps for large defects of the eyebrow, glabella, forehead and temple. Ophthal Plast Reconstr Surg 2002;18:138–145.)

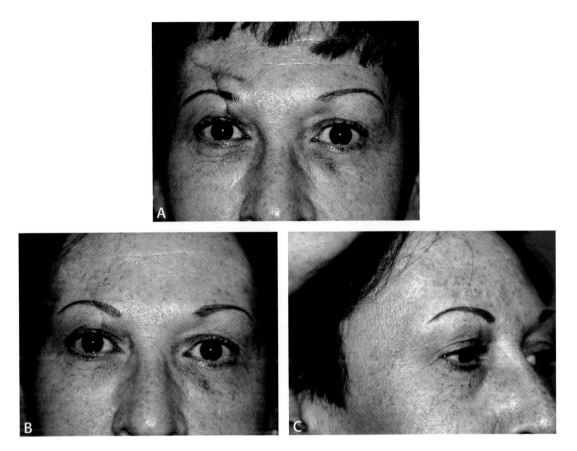

Figure 5.9

Postoperative appearance of patient depicted in Figure 5.8. **A.** Patient 7 weeks after surgery. **B, C.** Patient 5 months after surgery. Patients are forewarned that scars will be obvious for some time, but are also reassured that the long-term outcome will be preferable to that of a large, bulky flap. (Reproduced with permission from Lippincott Williams & Wilkins. Source: Harris GJ, Garcia GH. Advancement flaps for large defects of the eyebrow, glabella, forehead and temple. Ophthal Plast Reconstr Surg 2002;18:138–145.)

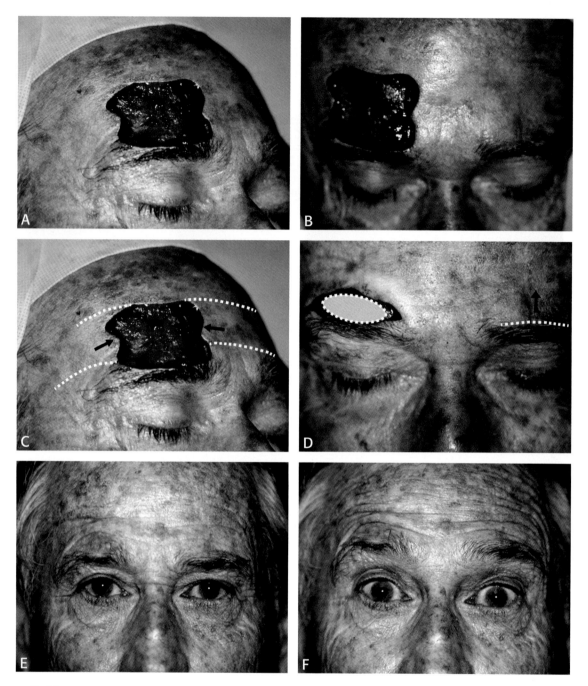

Figure 5.10

A, B. Broad defect of the forehead and upper portion of eyebrow. **C.** Primary repair with opposing advancement flaps. **D.** Mild right-brow retraction was addressed 3 months later with a small graft and a compensatory lift of the fellow eyebrow. **E, F.** Patient 6 months after the second procedure, with symmetry of eyebrow position and movement. (Grafted area is visible.) (Modified and reproduced with permission from Lippincott Williams & Wilkins. Source: Harris GJ, Garcia GH. Advancement flaps for large defects of the eyebrow, glabella, forehead and temple. Ophthal Plast Reconstr Surg 2002;18:138–145.)

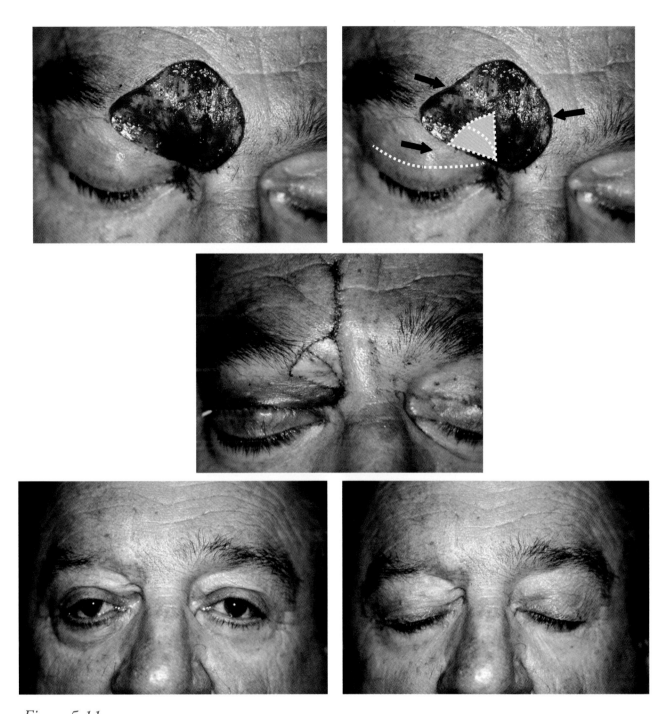

Figure 5.11

Large glabella/forehead/eyebrow/upper eyelid defect. Reconstruction involved direct advancement of the forehead and glabellar defect edges, a right upper eyelid advancement flap, and a supplemental postauricular skin graft (divided for fit). Although hair deficiency is obvious, the primary repair results are preferable to those with a midline forehead flap (see Fig. 5.1).

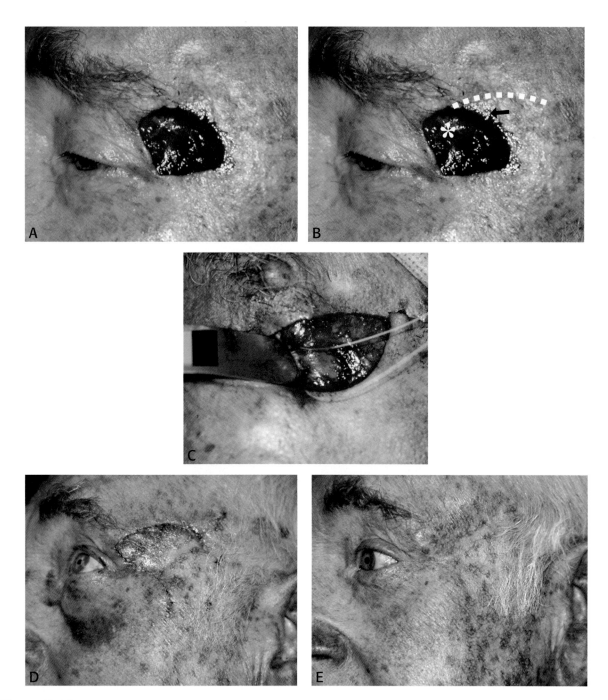

Figure 5.12

A, B. Defect of the lateral eyebrow and temple extending to the nonmarginal upper eyelid. To protect the loose eyelid skin from flap traction, the flap is anchored to periosteum (asterisk) over the lateral orbital rim. (See Chapter 3 for a discussion of anchored flaps in analogous defects of the cheek and lateral canthal sector.) **C.** The orbital septum is protected from the deep suture by a retractor against the rim (demonstrated in a similar case). **D.** Patient 1 week after surgery. **E.** Patient several months later.

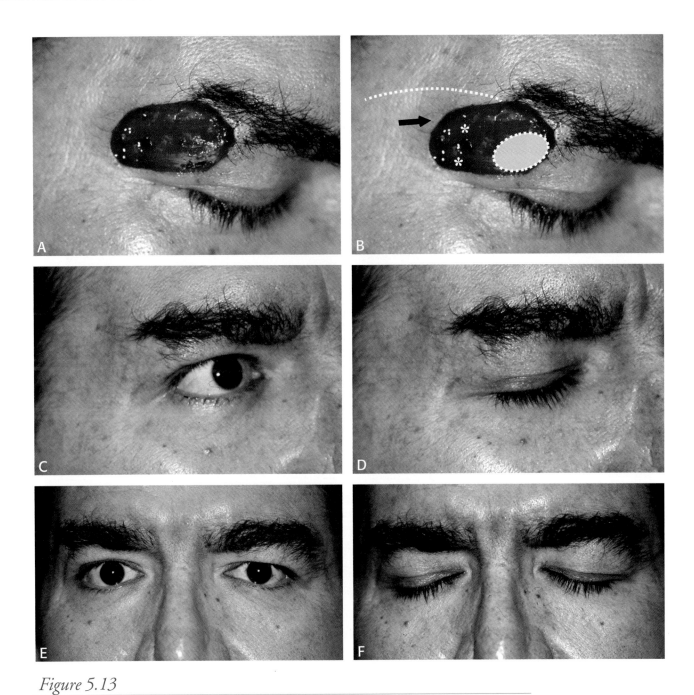

Figure 5.13

A, B. Defect of the lateral eyebrow and medial temple, with extension into the nonmarginal upper eyelid. Reconstruction included an advancement flap anchored at two sites on the orbital rim (asterisks), and a postauricular skin graft to the residual eyelid defect.
C–F. Patient 14 months after surgery.

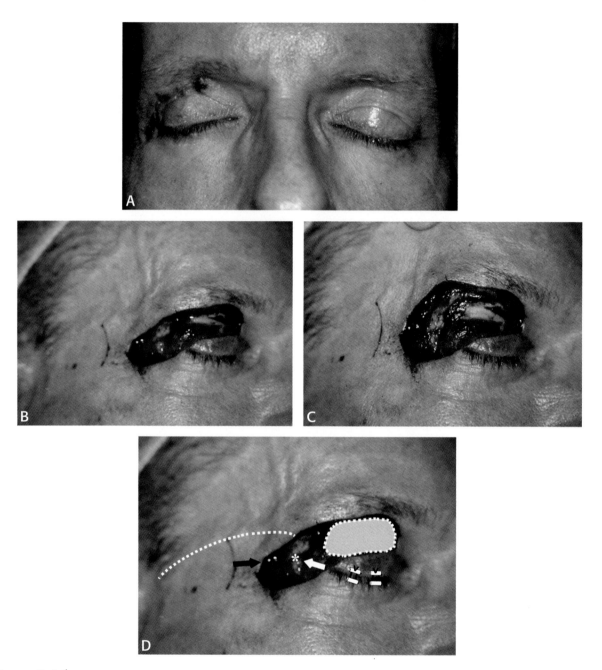

Figure 5.14

A. Long-standing basal cell carcinoma centered over the lateral orbital rim and extending toward the temple and well into the nonmarginal upper eyelid. The subbrow tissue was immobile. **B, C.** The post-Mohs defect included orbicularis muscle in all areas and portions of the orbital septum in the eyelid. Reconstructive requirements included thinner skin and greater mobility of the eyelid component, and thicker, more stable tissue laterally.
D. Reconstruction involved advancement and anchoring of a temporal flap over the lateral rim, tightening of the canthal attachment where the lateral raphe had been resected, a postauricular skin graft, and temporary tarsorrhaphies (5-0 polypropylene mattress sutures through silicone sponge bolsters) to counter the anticipated wound bed and skin graft contraction (see Fig. 5.15).

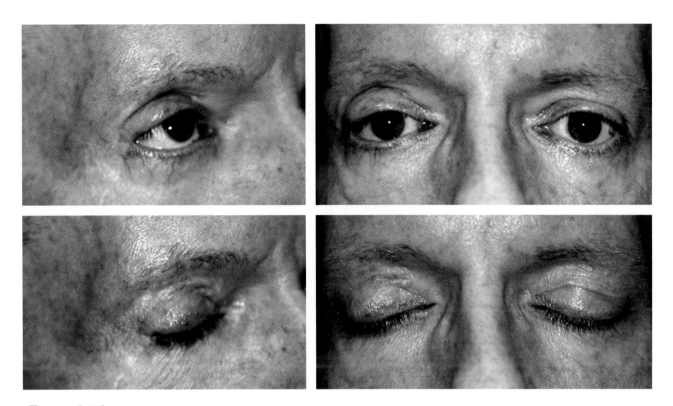

Figure 5.15

Patient 6 months after the surgery depicted in Figure 5.14.

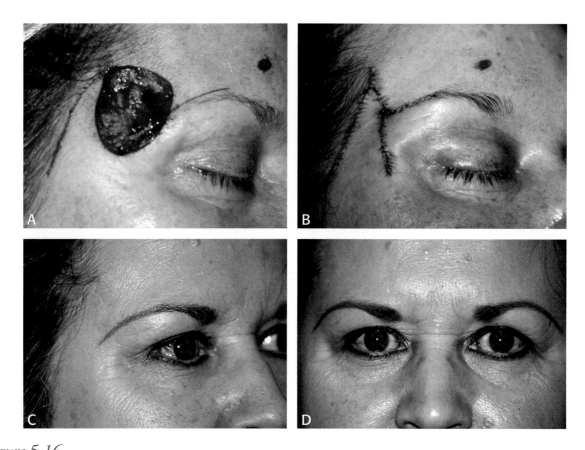

Figure 5.16

Large defect of the temple. **A, B.** Proximity of a defect to the hairline affects flap design. Flap alignment with subdermal apposition, however, is dictated by the direction of the eyebrow. Resulting superior and inferior redundancies are trimmed. Skin tension is moderate, but parallel to the brow. **C, D.** With time, the skin has stretched, eyebrow contour has normalized, and landmarks are preserved.

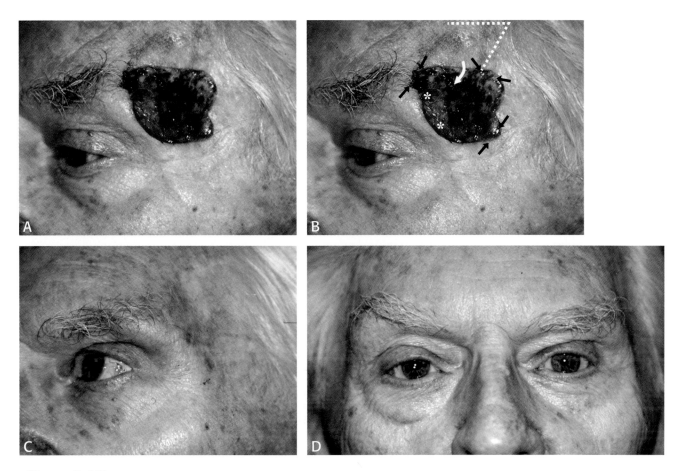

Figure 5.17

A. Defect of the lateral eyebrow and temple extending close to the hairline and over the lateral orbital rim. The patient's taut, sun-damaged skin and prior treatment of multiple facial skin cancers narrowed the options for flap design. **B.** Irregular corners were coapted with 6-0 nylon sutures, converting the defect to a near-rhomboid shape, and the rotation flap was then anchored to the orbital rim at two points (asterisks). **C, D.** Patient 9 months after surgery.

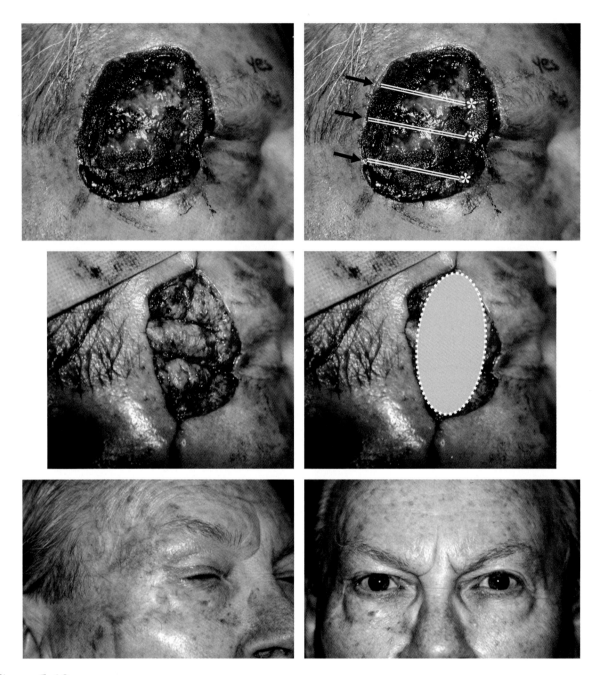

Figure 5.18

Large, shallow defect of the temple after staged resection of an in situ melanoma. Based on defect depth and size (relative to location and skin quality), grafting was chosen as the primary procedure. The defect, however, could be downsized with direct approximation superiorly and inferiorly, and with 4-0 subdermal polyglactin 910 sutures from the lateral edge to periosteum. This allowed a smaller (supraclavicular) full-thickness graft, and did not distort the canthus.

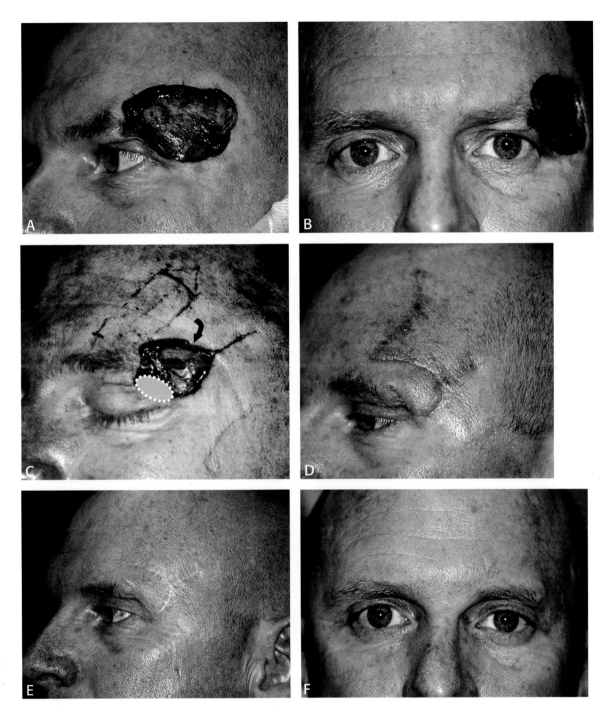

Figure 5.19

A, B. A large, deep defect involving the upper eyelid, eyebrow, forehead, and temple after Mohs resection of a squamous cell carcinoma with microscopic perineural invasion.
C. Based on defect depth and the anticipation of postoperative radiation, a well-vascularized flap was chosen as the primary reconstructive element. However, the defect could be downsized with direct approximation, allowing rotation of a smaller (Doppler-defined) axial forehead flap. A small skin graft resurfaced the subbrow defect. **D.** One-month result. **E, F.** Late, postradiation result.

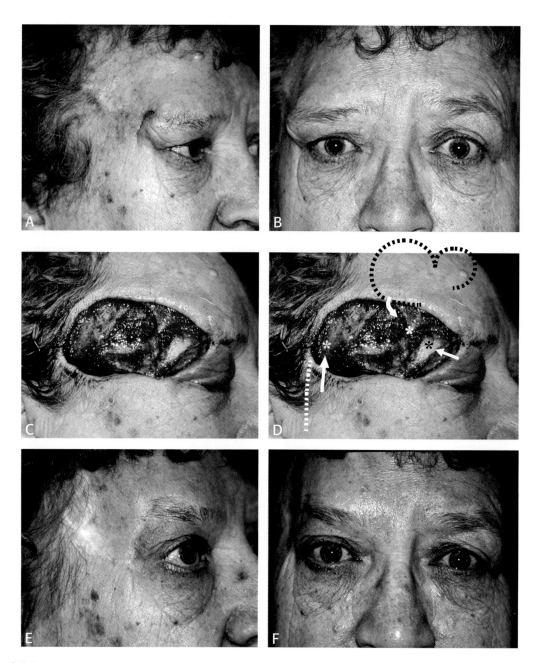

Figure 5.20

A, B. A 66-year-old woman with persistent basal cell carcinoma after multiple non-Mohs resections beginning 13 years earlier. **C.** Post-Mohs defect involving the eyebrow, temple, and forehead. Grafting was avoided because of defect depth. **D.** The medial edge was advanced over the bare orbital rim (black asterisk) and was anchored to a periosteal remnant, an inferior flap created with a pretrichial incision was advanced superiorly and anchored to deep temporal fascia (yellow asterisk), and a bilobed flap was rotated over exposed temporalis muscle and anchored to the posterior edge of the orbital rim (white asterisk). **E, F.** Patient 3 years after surgery. (Modified and reproduced with permission from Lippincott Williams & Wilkins. Source: Harris GJ, Garcia GH. Advancement flaps for large defects of the eyebrow, glabella, forehead and temple. Ophthal Plast Reconstr Surg 2002;18:138–145.)

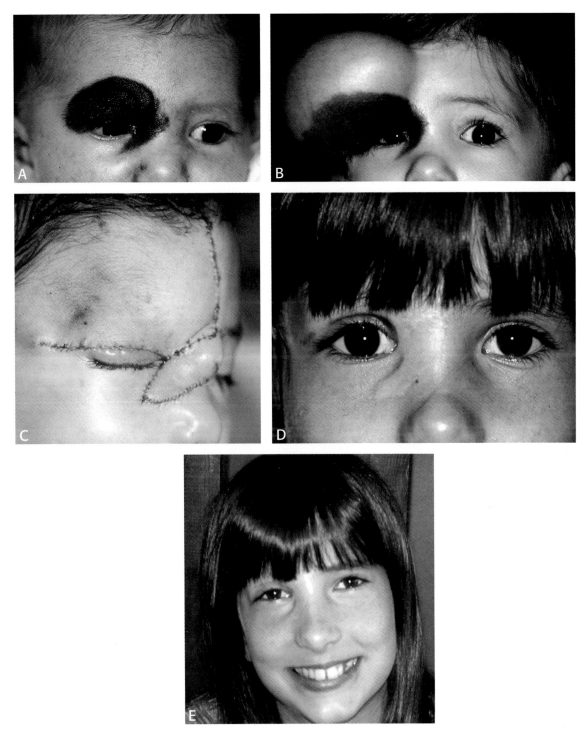

Figure 5.21

A. Infant with giant hairy nevus of nonmarginal upper eyelid, eyebrow, forehead, glabella, and medial canthus. **B.** Three months after placement of tissue expander, with incremental filling. **C.** Immediately after excision of lesion, removal of expander, and resurfacing of defect with expanded skin (medial aspect rotated to cover glabella and canthus). **D.** After pedicle excision. **E.** Patient 9 years after surgery. (Case managed jointly with Arun K. Gosain, MD.)

Reference

1. Harris GJ, Garcia GH. Advancement flaps for large defects of the eyebrow, glabella, forehead and temple. Ophthal Plast Reconstr Surg 2002;18:138–145.

6

Preoperative Counseling, Operative Protocol and Instruments, and Postoperative Management

*T*he procedures described in this text are primarily used after Mohs surgery, and although reconstructive techniques vary greatly with defect location, size, and complexity, there is relative uniformity in preoperative counseling, operative instrumentation and materials, and postoperative management.

Preoperative Consultation

After initial referral—generally by ophthalmologists for eyelid margin lesions and by dermatologists for more peripheral oculofacial lesions—patients undergo separate, tandem preoperative evaluations in the dermatologic surgery and oculoplastic surgery clinics. A full ophthalmologic examination is performed, and general medical history, medications, and allergies are reviewed. The reconstruction to be performed on the day of the scheduled surgery is broadly outlined. Although a range of procedures may be described, patients are advised that the precise techniques cannot be determined until the tumor-free defect has been created. I discuss the sector-specific risks (e.g., ectropion, canthal webbing, eyebrow distortion) that I expressly try to minimize, and I describe general differences between flaps and grafts. Patients are forewarned that they will have swelling and bruising for 7 to 10 days, that incisional scars will be most prominent at 4 to 6 weeks, and that progressive fading and improvement will continue for as long as 12 months. Some patients may be surprised at the attention given to lesions they had considered small and inconsequential. Candid preoperative discussion, however, can avert greater postoperative surprise and dissatisfaction if patients are unprepared for large defects, extensive reconstruction, or prolonged scar visibility.

Preoperative medical screening is performed by each patient's primary care physician, who has final discretion over suspending aspirin and anticoagulants. Although I prefer that clopidogrel (Plavix), aspirin, and nonsteroidal anti-inflammatory drugs be held for 5 days, and warfarin for 3 days, prior to reconstruction with flaps or grafts, recommendations are individualized for patients at high risk for life-threatening thromboembolic events.

Operative Protocol, Instruments, and Materials

Mohs micrographic surgery, using local infiltration anesthesia and including tissue processing and microscopic examination of specimens, is performed in the dermatologic surgery suite within the outpatient dermatology clinics. Lesions that require oculofacial reconstruction are usually removed during early-morning "first cases." After tumor-free margins have been confirmed, ophthalmic antibiotic ointment and sterile eye pads are applied. Patients are then transported by a family member to the outpatient ophthalmic surgery suite within the same medical complex. (Rarely, logistics require next-day reconstruction. The sterile eye pad is then maintained overnight, and an oral antibiotic is prescribed.)

An intravenous line is placed, and an anesthesiologist administers agents for sedation (e.g., midazolam) and analgesia (e.g., remifentanil, alfentanil, or fentanyl). In some cases, a sedative/hypnotic combination (e.g., propofol) or sedative/analgesic combination (e.g., ketamine) may be used. The dressing is removed and the defect is photographed. Using sterile technique around the fresh wound, prospective flaps are outlined with a marking pen, and local anesthetic (9:1 solution of 1% lidocaine with 1:100,000 epinephrine and 8.4% sodium bicarbonate) is injected through a half-inch 30-gauge needle. Regional (e.g., supraorbital, supratrochlear, infratrochlear, infraorbital) nerve blocks are used where appropriate, and prospective flaps are also infiltrated subcutaneously for hemostasis. After topical instillation of proparacaine, a full-face prep with 10% Betadine solution is performed. The entire face is left undraped, and a sterile nasal cannula is secured with half-inch Steri-Strips (Fig. 6-1). The nonoperative eye is covered with a gauze pad, and the operative eye is protected with a plastic eye shield. A 4-0 Mersilene traction suture is passed through the margin of the operative eyelid and secured with a mosquito hemostat.

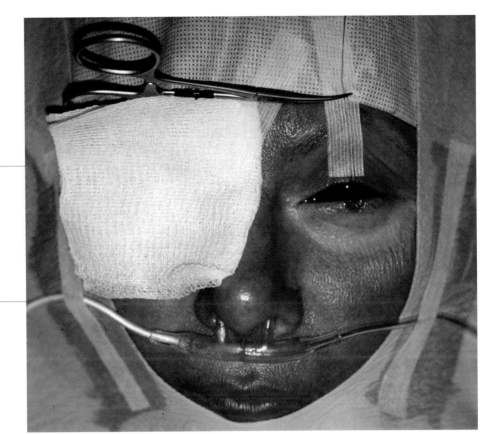

Figure 6-1

The entire face is prepped and included in the operative field. A sterilized nasal cannula is fixed to the benzoin-swabbed drape with half-inch Steri-Strips. A 4-0 Mersilene suture provides traction.

Surgical instruments are shown in Figure 6-2, and sutures and other materials are listed in Table 6-1. Tarsal remnants within marginal defects are "squared off" with a #15 Bard-Parker scalpel blade, 0.3-mm Castroviejo forceps, and sharp, pointed-tip, curved Westcott scissors. Using Castroviejo needleholders, eyelid margin edges are aligned with 6-0 black silk sutures, and tarsal and retractor edges are approximated with 6-0 polyglactin 910 sutures. Relaxing incisions for advancement or rotation flaps are made with #15 or #15C Bard-Parker blades, depending on the "tightness" of incision sites and curves. Flaps are elevated with Westcott scissors, while 0.12-mm and 0.3-mm Castroviejo forceps and small double skin hooks provide retraction. Hemostasis is maintained with bipolar cautery, using a fine, straight jewelers-tip forceps. Flaps are anchored to periosteum or medial canthal tendon with 4-0, 5-0, or 6-0 polyglactin 910 sutures, depending on flap thickness and tension. A narrow drain is placed beneath thin, broadly dissected flaps to prevent hematoma and seroma accumulation. A trimmed segment of a fluted silicone drain is used for this purpose, and it is fixed to the skin edge with a single 6-0 polyglactin 910 suture. Relaxing incisions are closed with continuous nylon sutures: 6-0 outside the orbital perimeter and 7-0

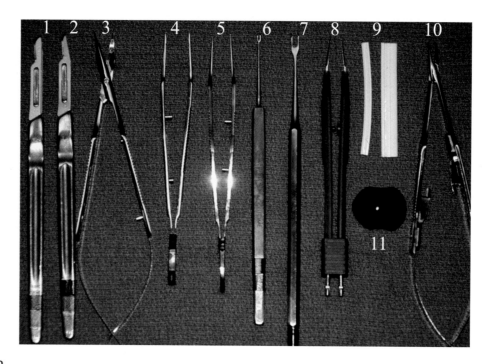

Figure 6-2

Surgical instruments used in oculofacial reconstruction. **1, 2.** Bard-Parker scalpel blades, #15 and #15C, respectively. **3.** Sharp, pointed-tip, curved Westcott scissors. **4, 5.** Castroviejo forceps, 0.3 mm and 0.12 mm, respectively. **6, 7.** Double skin hooks, small and medium, respectively. **8.** Nonstick, disposable bipolar forceps. **9.** Trimmed **(left)** and full-width **(right)** segments of a fluted, silicone Bard channel drain. **10.** Castroviejo needleholder. **11.** Plastic eye shield (scalloped edges reduce "suction cup" effect).

within it. Defect edges are apposed with subdermal 5-0, 6-0, or 7-0 polyglactin 910 sutures and cutaneous 6-0 or 7-0 nylon sutures, depending on edge thickness and wound tension. If there is oozing from the wound bed after closure has begun, topical thrombin is instilled beneath the flap through a cannula. A 7-0 nylon suture is placed through skin edges around the drain, but is not tied. The protective eye shield is removed, erythromycin ophthalmic ointment is applied, and a mild pressure dressing is placed. Patients are discharged and advised to keep their face dry overnight. Postoperative analgesics stronger than acetaminophen are rarely necessary.

Postoperative Management

Patients return for examination on the first postoperative day. The patch and drain are removed and the preplaced drain-site suture is tied. Patients are instructed to apply erythromycin ointment to sutures twice per day, to

Table 6-1

Sutures and Surgical Materials

BRAND NAME	MATERIAL	SIZE	NEEDLE	MANUFACTURER
Mersilene	Green braided polyester fiber suture	4-0	S-24	Ethicon, Inc., Somerville, NJ
Silk	Black braided silk suture	6-0	G-7	Ethicon, Inc., Somerville, NJ
Coated Vicryl Plus antibacterial with Ignacare	Undyed braided polyglactin 910 suture	4-0	TF	Ethicon, Inc., Somerville, NJ
Coated Vicryl Plus antibacterial with Ignacare	Undyed braided polyglactin 910 suture	5-0	P-2	Ethicon, Inc., Somerville, NJ
Coated Vicryl	Undyed braided polyglactin 910 suture	6-0	S-14	Ethicon, Inc., Somerville, NJ
Coated Vicryl	Violet, braided polyglactin 910 suture	7-0	TG 140-8	Ethicon, Inc., Somerville, NJ
Dermalon	Blue monofilament nylon suture	6-0	C-1	United States Surgical, Tyco Healthcare Group, LP, Norwalk, CT
Ethilon	Black monofilament nylon suture	7-0	P-6	Ethicon, Inc., Somerville, NJ
Bard-Parker Rib-Back	Carbon steel surgical blade	15, 15C	—	Becton Dickinson Acutecare, Franklin Lakes, NJ
Nonstick Disposable Bipolar Forceps	Jewelers/iris straight forceps	4 inch; 0.4-mm tip	—	Kirwan Surgical Products, Inc., Marshfield, MA
Bard Channel Drain	Silicone drain	7 mm, flat, 3/4 fluted	—	C. R. Bard, Inc., Covington, GA
Thrombin-JMI	Thrombin, topical U.S.P. (bovine origin)	5,000 IU vial	—	GenTrac, Inc., Middleton, WI
Steri-Strip	Sterile adhesive paper strips	0.5 inch	—	3M Health Care, St. Paul, MN
Harris Eye Shield	Scalloped, black plastic corneal protector	Small, medium, large	—	Eye Prosthetics of Wisconsin, Brookfield, WI
C-line Canaliculus Intubation Set	Silicone tubing (nylon-sheathed stainless steel stylettes)	33 cm long, 0.064 cm in diameter	—	Medtronic Xomed, Inc., Jacksonville, FL
Style #22 Silicone Button	Silicone button	4 × 5 mm	—	Labtician Ophthalmics, Inc., Oakville, ON

avoid excessive wetting, and not to apply ice or heat. If the reconstruction involved a skin graft or a thin, broadly dissected flap, patients are advised to avoid bending and heavy lifting.

Patients return for suture removal 6 to 8 days after surgery. They are advised to discontinue the ointment and to resume normal activity. They are also reminded that a mild increase in redness and induration of the incision sites during the following few weeks represents the normal wound-healing process.

At the 4- to 6-week postoperative visit, patients are reassured that scar prominence will gradually diminish over the ensuing months, and they are advised to apply vitamin E oil to nonmarginal incision sites twice per day.

Patients are seen 4 months after surgery to monitor scar prominence, and finally at 10 to 12 months after surgery to exclude local tumor recurrence. Annual full-body screening by a dermatologist is recommended thereafter. Scar revision or cosmetic touch-up procedures, such as thinning of a glabellar flap or Z-plasty revision of a medial canthal web, are not undertaken earlier than 1 year after the primary repair, and are performed in no more than 1% of cases.

Index

Note: Page numbers followed by *f* indicates figures; *t* indicates tables.